MEDICAL BOARDS STEP 1
made ridiculously simple

Andreas Carl, M.D., Ph.D.
Adjunct Assistant Professor
University of Nevada School of Medicine
Department of Physiology and Cell Biology
Reno, NV 89557-0046

MedMaster, Inc., Miami

ISBN #0-940780-52-6

Made in the United States of America

Published by
MedMaster, Inc.
P.O. Box 640028
Miami, FL 33164

For Dr. Anna Ivanenko.

This book would not have come to life without her
encouragement and enthusiasm.

PREFACE TO THE 3rd EDITION

With the new computerized testing, it is more important than ever to be able to relate the basic medical sciences you have learned in med school to clinical case presentations. I have significantly increased the amount of clinical correlations and placed each chart into a context. Hopefully, this will make "*Medical Boards Made Ridiculously Simple*" much more useful as a study tool, in addition to being a great "memory aid".

Your score on the USMLE Step 1 exam not only depends on how hard you study, but also what you study. Obviously, if you study what they ask, you can achieve a very high score. I have prepared this manuscript in order to help you maximizing your efforts. The material has been selected based on many years of teaching basic medical sciences to medical students and my own experience taking the USMLE Step 1. Recently there have been significant changes in the USMLE format and content and I wish to thank the many students whose input has allowed me to keep this book current and relevant for the USMLE exam.

Please visit my web-site to share your experiences with other students:

http://www.usmle.net

If you are about to take the exam or just took it, you can contact me via e-mail:

andreas@usmle.net

THE USMLE STEP 1 EXAM HAS BECOME SO CLINICAL IN NATURE, SHOULD I STUDY INTERNAL MEDICINE?

You will find that most exam questions are "wrapped" in a clinical case presentation, but in the end you still need to know the basic sciences in order to answer the questions. It is NOT necessary to know internal medicine to pass this exam (although it wouldn't hurt). Practically what this means for your test preparation is that you should focus on areas of basic science that have clear relevance to clinical medicine since these are much more likely to be made into a "case vignette" than some esoteric science facts. For this reason I have greatly increased the number of clinical comments and explanations for the 3rd edition of this book.

WHAT ARE HIGH-YIELD FACTS?

You need to know that what may be of high yield in one year could very well be of low yield the next year. There are some clear trends (emphasis of molecular biology, de-emphasis of gross anatomy) but with the random selection of questions by the testing computer, you cannot rely on "high-yield facts" alone. You must be able to place these into a practical context. The new edition of this book provides this context wherever possible.

WHY THE CHART FORMAT?

Well, I made these charts for myself when I took the USMLE and found it a fantastic memory-aid! Charts allow a more logical arrangement of basic science facts that can easily be build upon rather than just a random collection of materials. Studying in such systematic fashion lets you avoid the "high-yield trap". I have chosen the chart-format in order to provide the maximum amount of information with the minimum amount of words. By concentrating on key associations you will certainly improve your performance in multiple choice situations.

WHAT THIS BOOK IS NOT:

Medical Boards Made Ridiculously Simple is not a textbook and I recommend you use it side by side with your other review books. I have tried to be clear, comprehensive and very brief. It is not necessary to memorize the charts like a poem. As you become more familiar with the material, you should be able to read through the whole book within a few hours and develop a feeling of "déjà-vu".

HOW TO USE THIS BOOK?

This book is best used side by side with your other text and review books. You can "personalize" the charts by adding information that appears important or interesting to you. **The logical arrangement of basic science facts in charts will make it very easy to review all USMLE subjects just a few days before the exam.** I recommend reviewing the tables many times until they become boring. This is a good sign - meaning you recognize the stuff. It's not necessary to be able to actively reproduce the material given here, as long as you recognize the key associations in a "multiple choice situation".

> ➤ Use it during your course work to organize your thoughts
> ➤ Use it as a refresher course
> ➤ Use it as a last minute review

I wish to thank Steve Goldberg for the cartoons. Figures 4.29-4.38 were modified and reproduced with permission from Smith, L.H. and Thier, S.O. *Pathophysiology - The Biological Principles of Disease*. W.D. Saunders Co., 1985.

I hope that this text will help your preparation for the USMLE Step 1 and would appreciate any comments about the selection and presentation of this material you might have. Good luck!

PATHOLOGY

- This should be the center piece of your studies, it's also the most valuable for your future practice of medicine.

- Both Rubin and Farber's Pathology (16) and Robbins-Cotran (14) are excellent text books but too long for review. If you have used them during your class you may want to review the pictures and highlighted texts. The Board Review Series Pathology book by Schneider and Szanto (17) is highly recommended.

- Spend a day just looking at pictures, until you can recognize the most important ones (see "*hot pics*" at end of chapter 1), but don't go overboard – in many cases you will be able to answer the question from the case presentation alone, even if you don't recognize the picture.

- If you are ambitious, go over Compton's Review Questions (15). These are very difficult! If you get about 50% right, you should do very well on the Boards.

MICROBIOLOGY

- Just study them bug by bug, Levinson-Jawetz (13) is an excellent text.

- Also check out *Clinical Microbiology Made Ridiculously Simple* (6). This book contains over 200 cartoons which makes microbiology total fun.

- Know all the details, structure/function of the HIV virus. Study therapy of AIDS related infectious diseases.

- If you have time to spare, read "Immunology" from the NMS series (12). There are many questions on the exam, and this book covers it all.

PHARMACOLOGY

- Harvey-Champe (19) is "dead-on". If you know this book, you should get close to 100% right.

- *Clinical Pharmacology Made Ridiculously Simple* (8) contains a large number of tables comparing drugs side by side. Very complete! Excellent review, not just for the Boards but also for later.

- I found flash cards very useful. Make two sets: one for drug names versus mechanism of action and/or indication, and one set for drug names versus side effects. It is always best to make your own flash cards!!!

BIOCHEMISTRY

- Champe-Harvey (2) is "dead-on". If you know this book, you should get close to 100% right.

- In case you got lost, I recommend *Clinical Biochemistry Made Ridiculously Simple* (5) for a quick overview of the wondrous and amazing Land of Biochemistry.

ANATOMY

- Don't spend too much time on this subject. Best preparation is to look at pictures, including plenty of cross sections (CT or MRI scans) of the body.

- Read *Clinical Anatomy Made Ridiculously Simple* (4), but even this may be overkill.

- Read *Clinical Neuroanatomy Made Ridiculously Simple* (7). Read this one twice!

- Embryology and Histology are very minor subjects.

PHYSIOLOGY

- A difficult subject because you cannot memorize it. Even if you knew your Ganong (21) or Guyton (24), you may not be able to answer all questions. I very much like the *Color Atlas of Physiology* by Despopoulos and Silbernagel (9) for a quick review.

- Concentrate on kidneys, heart and lungs!
- A recent trend on the USMLE is receptors, signal transduction mechanisms and molecular biology of the cell.

SOCIAL SCIENCES

- Don't waste too much time here, but read *USMLE Behavioral Science Made Ridiculously Simple* (25). Some things you need to know very well are:

- Differences between normal grief reaction and adjustment disorders, neuroses and psychoses, dementia and delirium.
- Defense mechanisms.

- Sensitivity / Specificity / Negative predictive value etc. It's not enough to memorize what to divide by what, you need to understand the meaning of these.
- Design of clinical trials.
- Signs of child abuse.

PRACTICE QUESTIONS

- You will find the real exam very different from any collection of multiple choice questions or practice tests currently on the market. The real exam is more clinical in nature and questions tend to be longer. Don't panic - everyone is "in the same boat". There are retired board questions, but remember: they are retired for a reason! I found the *Pretest Questions* series more difficult than the actual board exam. The Appleton & Lange (1) and NMS questions (22) are a bit easier. Practice as many questions as possible.

- Don't use questions to "test" yourself. Don't be concerned about how many percent you get right. Mark all questions you get wrong with a pen, identify your areas of weakness and concentrate your studies on these. Later review just the questions you got wrong the first time and see how much you have learned.

- Don't practice multiple choice questions the week before the exam. You will get tired, bored and frustrated. Negative feelings might carry over to the exam day.

COMPUTER ADAPTIVE TESTING

- CAT is "around the corner", so how does it work? The computer will select questions based on your prior answers. If you get an answer wrong, the computer will choose an easier question, if you get the answer right, the computer will select a more difficult question. You need to know that this is a *statistical process* and you may find questions that are considered "difficult" easy, and questions that are considered "easy" more difficult; thus you probably will not be aware during the exam which direction the computer is going.

- The exam is terminated as soon as the computer reaches a statistical probability that you have passed or failed.

- Please visit www.usmle.org for news on computer adaptive testing!

ADVICE FOR FOREIGN MEDICAL GRADUATES

- It's especially important to get a good score the first time around since it has become more and more difficult for foreign medical graduates to get into a Residency program.

- Only 50% of foreign medical graduates pass on first attempt, compared to 95% of US and Canadian medical students. A major reason for this difference is language comprehension. Make sure you study from US review books since emphasis may be quite different from what you learned in your Country.

- Questions on the USMLE have become exceedingly long and you may struggle to finish in time. Practice as many questions as you can (at least 1,000). Make sure to practice some under "real-time" conditions: do 180 questions in 2½ hours without a break.

- It is useful to read the last sentence of each question first, then take a quick glance (no more!) at the answer choices, then go back and read the text of the question very selectively.

IMPORTANT

- Don't study any new material the day before the exam. It is more important to be well rested. For every fact you memorize on the day prior to the exam, you will lose some other one!

REFERENCES

1. A&L's Review for the USMLE Step 1, T.K. Barton, Appleton & Lange
2. Biochemistry, Champe & Harvey, Lippincott
3. Biochemistry, Stryer, Freeman
4. Clinical Anatomy Made Ridiculously Simple, S.Goldberg, MedMaster
5. Clinical Biochemistry Made Ridiculously Simple, S.Goldberg, MedMaster
6. Clinical Microbiology Made Ridiculously Simple, Gladwin & Trattler, MedMaster
7. Clinical Neuroanatomy Made Ridiculously Simple, S.Goldberg, MedMaster
8. Clinical Pharmacology Made Ridiculously Simple, J. Olson, MedMaster
9. Color-Atlas of Physiology, Despopoulos & Silbernagl, Thieme
10. Comprehensive Textbook of Psychiatry, Kaplan, Williams & Wilkin
11. Drug Evaluations, American Medical Association
12. Immunology, R.Hyde, Harwal Publishing
13. Medical Microbiology & Immunology, Levinson-Jawetz, Appleton & Lange
14. Pathologic Basis of Disease, Robbins & Cotran, Saunders
15. Pathologic Basis of Disease - Selfassessment and Review, Saunders
16. Pathology, Rubin & Farber, Lippincott
17. Pathology, Schneider & Szanto, Board Review Series, Williams & Wilkin
18. Pharmacologic Basis of Therapeutics, Goodman & Gilman, Macmillan
19. Pharmacology, Harvey & Champe, Lippincott
20. Physiological Basis of Medical Practice, J.B.West, Williams & Wilkin
21. Review of Medical Physiology, W.F. Ganong, Appleton & Lange
22. Review for USMLE Step 1, NMS, Williams & Wilkin
23. Sherris Medical Microbiology, K.J. Ryan, Appleton & Lange
24. Textbook of Medical Physiology, Guyton & Hall, Saunders
25. USMLE Behavioral Science Made Ridiculously Simple, F. Sierles, MedMaster

 CRCRCRCRCRCRCRCRCRCRCRCRCRCRCR

WHAT'S NEXT ?

You will need Chapters 1-3 (Pathology, Microbiology and Pharmacology) for a lightening fast review just prior to taking the Step 2 exam. My book *Medical Boards Step 2 Made Ridiculously Simple* will help you prepare for this exam but I have not repeated this information in the Step 2 book. It's always best to do your review from books and materials you already have mastered once.

CONTENTS

TABLE OF CONTENTS

PATHOLOGY

A) GENERAL PATHOLOGY

B) ORGAN PATHOLOGY

MICROBIOLOGY

A) GENERAL MICROBIOLOGY

B) BACTERIA

BIOCHEMISTRY

ANATOMY

A) EMBRYOLOGY

B) GROSS ANATOMY

C) NEUROANATOMY

PHYSIOLOGY

SOCIAL SCIENCES

A) PSYCHOLOGY

B) PSYCHOPATHOLOGY

C) STATISTICS

PATHOLOGY

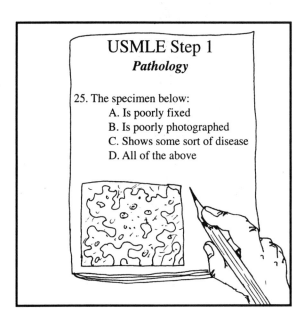

USMLE Step 1
Pathology

25. The specimen below:
   A. Is poorly fixed
   B. Is poorly photographed
   C. Shows some sort of disease
   D. All of the above

Part A : General Pathology

1.1.) INFLAMMATION

> red'n tender – warm'n swollen

Acute inflammation is the response of tissue to any kind of damage. It is non-specific, allows immune cells to access the damaged area and clear away dead tissues.

ACUTE INFLAMMATION:
- increased blood flow
- increased vascular permeability
- emigration of leukocytes

MEDIATORS OF INFLAMMATION:

fever	IL-1, prostaglandins
vasodilatation	nitric oxide prostaglandins
exudation	histamine, bradykinin
chemotaxis	complement C5a, IL-8
phagocytosis	complement C3b (opsonin)
pain	prostaglandins, bradykinin

Which parts of the inflammatory response depend on prostaglandins? Can you see how inhibitors of prostaglandin synthesis like aspirin alleviate many symptoms of inflammation (fever, swelling, pain) but not necessarily the inflammatory process itself?

1.2.) <u>CYTOKINES</u>

<u>There is lots of overlap and redundancy:</u>
- cytokines have a wide spectrum of effects.
- each cytokines may be produced by several cell types.
- each leukocyte produces several cytokines.

<u>MAIN FUNCTIONS OF CYTOKINES</u>:

during acute inflammation (produced by phagocytes)	IL-1, IL-8, TNF-α
activators of lymphocytes	**T-cells:** IL-1 **B-cells:** IL-2, IL-4, IL-5

Cytokines orchestrate the immune response. It is an almost hopeless task to list <u>all</u> interactions between cells during an inflammatory process. Some of the major ones you may want to know:

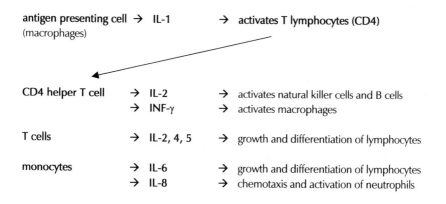

antigen presenting cell →	IL-1	→	activates T lymphocytes (CD4)
(macrophages)			

CD4 helper T cell	→ IL-2	→ activates natural killer cells and B cells
	→ INF-γ	→ activates macrophages
T cells	→ IL-2, 4, 5	→ growth and differentiation of lymphocytes
monocytes	→ IL-6	→ growth and differentiation of lymphocytes
	→ IL-8	→ chemotaxis and activation of neutrophils

MAJOR CYTOKINES:

		PRODUCED BY:	ACTION:
A)	α-interferon	leukocytes	- antiviral - induces **MHC-I** expression
	β-interferon	fibroblasts	- antiviral - induces **MHC-I** expression
	γ-interferon	T cells	- activates macrophages - induces **MHC-II** expression *(on macrophages)*
B)	IL-1	macrophages	**fever**
	IL-2, IL-3, IL-4, IL-5	T cells	activates many other cells
	IL-6	macrophages fibroblasts	activates many other cells
	IL-7	bone marrow cells	activates many other cells
C)	TNF-α	macrophages	like IL-1
D)	PDGF	platelets endothelial cells	**proliferation of vascular smooth muscle cells**

Mutation of IL-2 receptor is the cause of severe combined immune deficiency!

1.3.) <u>COMPLEMENT</u>

Complement proteins are enzymes that form a cascade, directed at cleavage of C3. The common final pathway leads to formation of the membrane attack complex. Activation of the alternative pathway does not require specific antibodies (i.e. previous sensitization) but contact with yeast, bacterial cell walls or endotoxins:

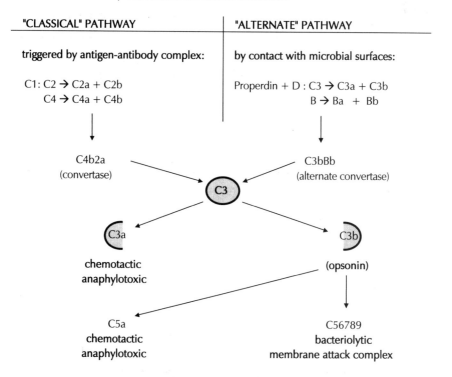

"CLASSICAL" PATHWAY | "ALTERNATE" PATHWAY

triggered by antigen-antibody complex: | by contact with microbial surfaces:

C1: C2 → C2a + C2b | Properdin + D : C3 → C3a + C3b
C4 → C4a + C4b | B → Ba + Bb

C4b2a | C3bBb
(convertase) | (alternate convertase)

C3

C3a | C3b
chemotactic | (opsonin)
anaphylotoxic

C5a | C56789
chemotactic | bacteriolytic
anaphylotoxic | membrane attack complex

Complement activity can be measured and is used clinically to follow SLE or immune complex diseases.

1.4.) <u>AUTOANTIBODIES</u>

rheumatoid arthritis	anti-IgG (rheumatoid factor)
systemic lupus	anti-nuclear antibodies (ANA)
drug induced lupus	anti-histone
CREST	anti-centromere
myasthenia gravis	anti-ACh receptor
Graves' disease	anti-TSH receptor
Hashimoto's thyroiditis	anti-microsomal
Wegener's granulomatosis	anti-neutrophil cytoplasm (ANCA)
primary biliary cirrhosis	anti-mitochondrial
celiac sprue	anti-gliadin
Goodpasture's syndrome	anti glomerular basement membrane

1.5.) <u>WHAT IS AMYLOID?</u>

- *amorphous, eosinophilic <u>extracellular</u> substance*
- *consists of fibril protein and glycoprotein*
- *Congo-Red stain → green birefringence under polarizing microscope*
  (this distinguishes amyloid from other hyaline deposits: collagen, fibrin…)

<u>There are 2 types of amyloid:</u>
AL: Amyloid light chains ← multiple myeloma
AA: Amyloid associated protein ← chronic inflammation and aging

1.6.) <u>HYPERSENSITIVITY</u>

	MEDIATORS	SIGNS & SYMPTOMS	EXAMPLES
Type I IgE	- mast cells - basophils → histamine	urticaria erythema bronchiole constriction laryngeal edema shock, death	**anaphylaxis** **asthma** hay fever eczema
Type II IgG, IgM	antibodies bind to cell surface and activate complement	hemolysis	**transfusion reaction** drug reactions erythroblastosis fetalis autoimmune diseases
Type III IgM, IgG	immune complexes get deposited and activate complement	urticaria lymphadenopathy arthritis vasculitis glomerulonephritis	**serum sickness** Arthus reaction
Type IV	T cells (memory cells) activate macrophages and killer cells resulting in cell damage.	erythema with induration	**tuberculin reaction** "delayed hypersensitivity"

Serum sickness: nowadays mostly caused by drugs.
Arthus reaction: edema and necrosis following intradermal injection of drugs.

TRANSPLANT REJECTION:
Hyperacute: due to preformed antibodies.
Acute: mostly due to type IV reaction.

1.7.) <u>ONCOGENES</u>

	GENE PRODUCT	DISEASE
c-myc	transcription factor	Burkitt lymphoma
c-abl	tyrosine kinase	CML
bcl-2	inhibits apoptosis	Non-Hodgkin lymphoma
ras	G protein	colon carcinoma

<u>What activates oncogenes ?</u>
1. Chromosomal rearrangement brings dormant oncogene next to a promoter.
2. Mutations.

1.8.) <u>TUMOR SUPPRESSOR GENES</u>

	DISEASE
RB1	• retinoblastoma
BRCA-1	• breast cancer • ovarian cancer
p53	• breast carcinoma • colon carcinoma • bronchial carcinomas

Tumors sometimes develop several oncogen/suppressor gene abnormalities and become more aggressive.

1.9.) TUMOR MARKERS

Tumor markers are used for follow-up after treatment to detect metastases, but not for screening an asymptomatic population.

CEA	• adenocarcinomas (colon, pancreas, lung)
alpha-fetoprotein	• hepatoma • twin pregnancy • anencephalus
PSA	• prostate carcinoma • more sensitive than acid phosphatase
acid phosphatase	• prostate carcinoma
alkaline phosphatase	• metastases to bones • obstructive biliary disease • Paget's disease

1.10.) METASTASES

Knowing which tumors form metastases where is important:
Sometimes you find the metastasis first and must search for the primary!

	MOST COMMON PRIMARY SITE
brain	lung > breast
bone	breast > lung
liver	colon > stomach > pancreas

1.11.) GENETICS - PEDIGREES

AUTOSOMAL DOMINANT: (vertical pattern)

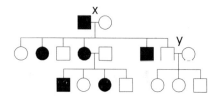

X: Sick person marries healthy one: 50% of children will be sick
                                                      males and females have equal risk

Y: Healthy child marries healthy persons: 100% normal offspring

Every sick person has at least one sick parent!

AUTOSOMAL RECESSIVE: (horizontal pattern)

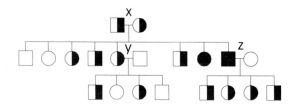

X: If two heterozygotes marry: 25% children will be normal
                                                     50% children will be heterozygous
                                                     25% children will be sick

Y: Heterozygote marries healthy: 50% children will be normal
                                                     50% children will be heterozygous
                                                     0% children will be sick

Z: Homozygote marries healthy: 100% children will be heterozygous

X-LINKED RECESSIVE: (oblique pattern)

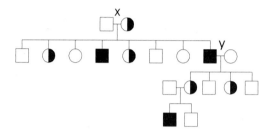

X: Carrier marries healthy male: 50% sons will be sick
50% sons will be healthy
100% daughters will be healthy
50% daughters will be carriers

Y: Sick male marries healthy female: all sons will be healthy
all daughters will be carriers

Disease tends to skip generations!
Male to male transmission of disease rules out X-linked disease!

☐   healthy male
○   healthy female
■   sick male
●   sick female
◖   heterozygote (carrier)

You should be able to recognize these patterns. Do not memorize the % numbers, try to figure them out yourself from the chromosomal distribution!

1.12.) <u>AUTOSOMAL RECESSIVE DISEASES</u>

cystic fibrosis	pulmonary infections chronic pancreatitis
phenylketonuria	fair skin, blue eyes mental retardation if untreated
albinism	sunburn, squamous carcinoma of skin
α1-antitrypsin deficiency	emphysema, liver cirrhosis
thalassemias, sickle cell anemias	anemia
glycogen storage diseases	affects liver, muscles, heart (plus hypoglycemia in some)
mucopolysaccharidoses (except Hunter's)	lysosomal storage disease: - facial deformities - mental and physical retardation
sphingolipidoses (except Fabry's)	lysosomal storage disease: - hepatomegaly, splenomegaly
polycystic kidney disease (infant type)	kidney failure
hemochromatosis	liver cirrhosis, diabetes cardiac failure
Chédiak-Higashi syndrome	bacterial and fungal infections of skin and mucous membranes due to impaired leukocyte function

 Albinism: *Melanocytes are present but contain only unpigmented melanosomes.*

1.13.) <u>AUTOSOMAL DOMINANT DISEASES</u>

familial hypercholesterolemia	abnormal LDL receptor coronary artery disease
familial polyposis	colon cancer
spherocytosis	hemolytic anemia
von Willebrand disease	bleeding
Ehlers-Danlos syndrome	stretchy skin sprains, joint dislocations
Marfan syndrome	long bones lens dislocation
achondroplasia	premature ossification dwarfism: short limbs, normal trunk
phacomatoses	benign tumors of eye, skin and brain
Huntington's disease	chorea dementia
polycystic kidney disease (adult type)	kidney failure

 Please compare the 2 types of polycystic kidney disease:

ADULT TYPE	INFANT TYPE
• common • dominant	• rare • recessive
• berry aneurysms	• liver cysts

1.14.) X-LINKED RECESSIVE DISEASES

hemophilia A and B	bleeding
glucose-6-phosphate deficiency	hemolytic anemia
fragile X	mild mental retardation
Fabry disease	sphingolipidosis - cardiomegaly - angiokeratoma
Lesch-Nyhan syndrome	self mutilation + gout
Duchenne	muscle dystrophy – absent dystrophin
Becker	muscle dystrophy – aberrant dystrophin
Bruton's agammaglobulinemia	low or absent B cells
Wiskott-Aldrich syndrome	functional deficiency of B and T cells thrombocytopenia
chronic granulomatous disease	defect of neutrophil free radical formation

Female carriers of X-linked disorders are rarely affected because of the random inactivation of one of the X chromosomes in every cell (Lyon hypothesis).

Fragile X chromosome:
Fragile "knob" connected by a stalk to the main part of chromosome X which breaks off easily during karyotyping.
- Female carriers of fragile X may have slight mental retardation.
- Some affected males are mentally normal.

1.15.) <u>DELETIONS</u>

Deletion of an entire autosomal chromosome is not compatible with life !

PARTIAL DELETIONS:

5p	cri du chat syndrome (newborn infants cry like kittens)
11p	congenital absence of iris
13q	retinoblastoma

p: short arm of chromosome

q: long arm of chromosome

VERY CURIOUS CASE:

Prader Willi syndrome	15q11-13 deletion (paternal chromosome) • severe infantile hypotony • obesity • mental retardation
Angelman syndrome	15q11-13 deletion (maternal chromosome) • "happy puppet" syndrome • happy smile, wide-based gait • epilepsy

It's a mystery! Why does a deletion of the maternally versus paternally derived chromosome 15 cause such a different phenotype?

1.16.) <u>HLA</u>

Some major histocompatibility antigens predispose to getting disease:

A3	• hemochromatosis
B27	• ankylosing spondylitis • Reiter's syndrome • ulcerative colitis
DR2	• multiple sclerosis • narcolepsy
DR3	• SLE • IDDM
DR4, Dw4, Dw14	• rheumatoid arthritis • juvenile rheumatoid arthritis

---

RBC antigens are "naturally occurring" antigens:
Patients form antibodies against those antigens they do not possess.

Leukocyte antigens are not "naturally occurring":
Patients do not form antibodies unless sensitized (transplants)

Class I	Class II
• HLA-A, HLA-B, HLA-C	• HLA-D
• found on all cell surfaces	• found mostly on B-lymphocytes

1.17.) <u>MOST COMMON CAUSES</u>

A) <u>MALIGNANCIES</u>:

	INCIDENCE	MORTALITY
men	prostate > lung > colon	lung > prostate > colon
women	breast > lung > colon	lung > breast > colon

 Skin cancers are the most common malignancies, but usually ignored from statistics because of their low mortality.

MALIGNANCIES IN CHILDREN:

Most common malignancy **overall**:	leukemia (ALL)
Most common **solid** malignancy:	brain tumors
Most common solid malignancy **outside CNS**:	neuroblastoma

B) <u>OTHER DISEASES</u>:

acute renal failure	tubular necrosis
nephrotic syndrome	**children:** minimal change glomerulonephritis **adults:** membranous glomerulonephritis
nephritic syndrome	poststreptococcal glomerulonephritis
hypertension	"idiopathic" ("essential" = we don't know the cause)
anemia	iron deficiency
amenorrhea	pregnancy
chronic pancreatitis	alcoholism
food poisoning	*Clostridia perfringens* *Staph. aureus* toxin

Part B : Organ Pathology

1.18.) <u>SLE</u>

ANA :	sensitive but not specific
anti ds-DNA and anti Sm :	specific but not sensitive

CLINICAL FEATURES OF SLE:

<u>SKIN</u>
- o Malar rash - spares nasolabial folds
- o Photosensitivity

<u>ORGANS</u>
- o Arthritis
- o Pleuritis
- o Pericarditis
- • Renal disease – proteinuria

<u>BLOOD</u>
- o Hemolytic anemia
- o Leukopenia
- o Lymphocytopenia

<u>LAB</u>
- ➤ Antinuclear antibodies
- ➤ False positive VDRL (cardiolipin antibodies)
- ➤ confirmed by negative FTA-ABS

__What is an LE cell ?__
Artificially injured leukocytes are mixed with patient's
macrophages. Macrophages then phagocytose nuclei of injured
leukocytes if the patient has SLE.

1.19.) <u>SYSTEMIC SCLEROSIS</u>

excessive fibrosis throughout the body

FEATURES	ANTIBODIES
a) limited = CREST localized scleroderma (fingers, forearm, face)	anti-centromere
b) diffuse systemic widespread scleroderma rapid progression early visceral involvement	anti-Scl 70 (topoisomerase I)

C alcinosis
R aynaud's
E sophageal dysmotility
S clerodactyly
T elangiectasis

1.20.) <u>SJÖGREN'S SYNDROME</u>

immunological destruction of salivary and lacrimal glands

FEATURES	ANTIBODIES
dry eyes, dry mouth	**SS-A** (anti Ro) **SS-B** (anti La)

1.21.) IMMUNODEFICIENCIES

Pay close attention to the clinical features - you can make a diagnostic guess based on the clinical presentation alone:

			CLINICAL FEATURES:
severe combined	lymphopenia (B and T)	X-linked or autosomal	death within first year
DiGeorge's	T cells absent	sporadic	viral infections fungal infections tetany
Bruton's	B cells absent	X-linked	bacterial infections
common variable	B cells present but produce few antibodies	variable	bacterial infections
IgA deficiency	low IgA	autosomal	sinopulmonary infections gastrointestinal infections
Wiskott-Aldrich	low IgM	X-recessive	bacterial infections thrombocytopenia eczema

- most common congenital immunodeficiency: IgA deficiency
- most common acquired immunodeficiency: AIDS

1.22.) <u>BLEEDING DISORDERS</u>

A) The most common <u>inherited</u> bleeding disorder is VonWillebrand's.

B) The most common <u>acquired</u> bleeding disorder is vitamin K deficiency.

		KEY FEATURES
A)	lack of factor VIII-R (Von Willebrand disease)	• aPTT prolonged • **bleeding time prolonged**
	lack of factor VIII (hemophilia A)	• aPTT prolonged • normal bleeding time
	lack of factor IX (hemophilia B)	• aPTT prolonged • normal bleeding time
B)	Vit. K deficiency (affects factors II, V, VII, IX, X)	• PT prolonged • fat malabsorption • antibiotics (diminished gut flora) • coumarin therapy
	ITP (idiopathic thrombocytic purpura)	• immune mediated • children: acute (post viral infection) • adults: often chronic
	TTP (thrombotic thrombocytic purpura)	• young women • microthrombi • fragmented RBCs (helmet cells)

Which disorders result in prolonged bleeding time and which do not? Why?

	<u>depends on:</u>
Bleeding Time:	platelet function
PT:	extrinsic + common pathways
aPTT:	intrinsic + common pathways
TT:	common pathway

1.23.) HEMOLYTIC ANEMIAS

Anemia results when the bone marrow cannot keep up with the shortened red blood cell survival (normal lifespan of RBC is ~120 days).

A) HEREDITARY:

	KEY FEATURES
spherocytosis	• autosomal dominant • defective spectrin • splenomegaly
G6PD deficiency	• hemolysis during oxidative stress such as: • viral infections, fava beans, • sulfa drugs, quinine, nitrofurantoin • Heinz bodies (=hemoglobin degradation products)
sickle cell anemia	HbS $(\alpha_2\beta^s_2)$ • sickling triggered by: hypoxia, dehydration, acidosis • vaso-occlusive crisis • aplastic crisis • sequestration crisis (splenomegaly) • autosplenectomy
α-Thalassemias	HbH (β_4) • common in Southeast Asia • hypochromic cells, target cells • Hb Bart (γ_4) → hydrops fetalis
β-Thalassemias[1]	HbA$_2$ $(\alpha_2\delta_2)$ and HbF $(\alpha_2\gamma_2)$ • common in Mediterranean and US • hypochromic cells, target cells

[1] **major** = homozygote, **minor** = heterozygote

ROLE OF SPLEEN:
Phagocytes of the spleen remove even slightly abnormal RBCs or RBCs covered with antibodies. However, "therapeutic splenectomy" is NOT beneficial!

B) IMMUNE MEDIATED:

warm antibodies (usually IgG)	cold antibodies (usually IgM)
active at 37°C	most active at 0~4°C
• drugs • malignancies • SLE	• mycoplasma pneumonia • mononucleosis • lymphoma

Cold antibodies*: Agglutination occurs only in peripheral cool
parts of the body → vascular obstruction → Raynaud's phenomenon.*

COOMBS TEST:

direct test: detects cell bound antibodies
(mix patient's RBCs with anti-IgG)

indirect test: detects free antibodies
(mix patient's plasma with normal RBCs)

1.24.) <u>OTHER ANEMIAS</u>

C) <u>INSUFFICIENT PRODUCTION:</u>

	KEY FEATURES
megaloblastic	• hypochromic, macrocytic RBCs • hypersegmented neutrophils • **folate** : anemia, no neurological symptoms • **B12** : anemia plus neurological symptoms
iron deficiency	• hypochromic, microcytic RBCs • chronic blood loss
aplastic (bone marrow failure)	• viral infections • toxins • drugs : alkylating agents chloramphenicol

In elderly patients with iron deficiency anemia you should always suspect a colorectal malignancy!

PLUMMER-VINSON: 1. anemia
2. atrophic glossitis
3. esophageal webs

FANCONI ANEMIA: 1. hypoplastic thumbs
(autosomal recessive)   2. absent radii
3. aplastic anemia
(bone marrow DNA is more susceptible to radiation and alkylating agents)

1.25.) RED BLOOD CELLS

If you discover RBCs with "special features" under the microscope,
an instant diagnosis can be made:

Heinz bodies (denatured hemoglobin)	• G6PD deficiency
Howell-Jolly bodies (nuclear fragments)	• post splenectomy
basophil stippling	• lead poisoning
siderocytes	• iron overload • Pappenheimer bodies
reticulocytes (remains of ribosomal RNA)	• increased production/release of RBCs • recovery from hemorrhage

RETICULOCYTE INDEX:
Following acute blood loss, the reticulocyte count may double within first
24h. It is important to relate the reticulocyte count to hematocrit in order
to correct for the blood loss (so called "reticulocyte index").

1.26.) <u>NEUTROPENIA</u>

decreased production	• megaloblastic anemia • some leukemias, lymphomas
increased destruction	• immune mediated (Felty's syndrome)
drug induced	• alkylating agents • chloramphenicol • chlorpromazine • sulfonamides • phenylbutazone

1.27.) <u>LEUKOCYTOSIS</u>

neutrophils	• acute infections • stress
eosinophils	• allergy, asthma • parasitic infections
lymphocytes	• tuberculosis • viral infections
monocytes	• tuberculosis • malaria • rickettsia

 Comparing Charts 1.26 and 1.27 – which is more alarming, leukopenia or leukocytosis?

1.28.) LEUKEMIAS

ALL	AML	CML	CLL	hairy cell leukemia
children	any age	young adults	elderly	
fever petechiae ecchymoses CNS infiltrate	fever petechiae ecchymoses lymphadenopathy (splenomegaly)	fever night sweats splenomegaly	insidious few symptoms low Ig levels infections	hepatomegaly splenomegaly
prognosis : good	depending on type	poor	fair	poor
lymphoblasts	Auer rods in myeloblasts	Philadelphia chro.	lymphocytes predominate	pancytopenia TRAP

PHILADELPHIA CHROMOSOME: (if present → better prognosis)
- c-abl proto-oncogene on chromosome 9 when translocated to the breakpoint region (bcr) of chromosome 22 forms a fusion gene (bcr/abl).
- This gene encodes a protein with high tyrosine kinase activity.

1.29.) LYMPHOMAS

HODGKIN'S DISEASE	NON-HODGKIN LYMPHOMAS
• spreads in contiguity • no leukemic component • Reed-Sternberg cells	• does not spread in contiguity • often has leukemic component • more common recently !!!

 Reed-Sternberg cells: *Nobody knows where these cells come from! They are binucleated, have prominent nucleoli and clear parachromatin.*

A) SUBTYPES HODGKIN:

	KEY FEATURES
a) lymphocyte predominance b) nodular sclerosis	these have better prognosis
c) mixed cellularity d) lymphocyte depletion	many Reed Sternberg cells → poor prognosis

B) SUBTYPES NON-HODGKIN:

"many subtypes, several classifications, lots of confusion"

CLASS	EXAMPLE
low grade (good prognosis)	small lymphocytic lymphoma
intermediate grade	large cell lymphoma
high grade (poor prognosis)	immunoblastic lymphoma Burkitt lymphoma

---

"Starry sky" pattern of Burkitt lymphoma:
the "stars": benign macrophages
the "sky": matrix of rapidly proliferating neoplastic B cells

---

1.30.) PLASMA CELL NEOPLASIAS

Myeloma is a plasma cell neoplasm that often presents as a "bone tumor".

MONOCLONAL GAMMOPATHY	MULTIPLE MYELOMA	WALDENSTRÖM'S
benign	malignant	malignant
usually IgG or IgA	usually IgG or IgA	always IgM
<10% plasma cells in bone marrow	"myeloma cells" (>10% plasma cells infiltrating bone)	"flame cells" (eosinophilic plasma cells)
may convert to multiple myeloma	osteoclast activating factor (→ "punched-out" skull, pelvis, etc.)	hyperviscosity syndrome
	Bence-Jones proteins amyloidosis (tissue deposit of λ-chains)	

M-PROTEIN:
- Monoclonal immunoglobulin secreted by a single clone of aberrant plasma cells.
- May be IgG, IgM etc.

BENCE-JONES PROTEIN:
- Excess light chains (due to unbalanced synthesis of immunoglobulins)
- These are readily filtered through the glomeruli and appear in urine.

1.31.) <u>PHLEBOTHROMBOSIS</u>

Risk factors:	- endothelial injury
	- slow blood flow
	- hypercoagulability
Trousseau's sign:	- migratory venous thrombosis
	- a/w neoplasms

 Pulmonary embolism is a major cause of death in the US. Most thrombi originate in the deep veins of the legs and risk factors are the same as for phlebothrombosis.

1.32.) <u>ARTERIOSCLEROSIS</u>

The pathologist distinguishes 4 types of arteriosclerosis depending on location and features:

	KEY FEATURES
atherosclerosis	• large and medium size arteries • fatty streaks • atheromas
Mönckeberg's	• media calcific stenosis • "gooseneck lumps" • small and medium size arteries • asymptomatic
arteriolosclerosis (hyperplastic)	• fibrinoid necrosis • malignant hypertension • "onion skin" hyperplasia
arteriolosclerosis (hyaline)	• diabetes mellitus • thickened basement membrane

1.33.) ARTERITIS

Try to memorize which vessels are affected by which diseases:

	KEY FEATURES
hypersensitivity arteritis	• small vessels • lesions all at same stage • cryoglobulins • a/w Henoch-Schönlein purpura
polyarteritis nodosa	• small and medium vessels • kidneys, heart, muscles, skin • can be fatal but responds well to steroids
thromboangiitis obliterans (Buerger's)	• small and medium vessels • in smokers
giant cell arteritis	temporal artery • sudden blindness • female > male • a/w polymyalgia rheumatica
Wegener's	• upper respiratory vasculitis • lower respiratory vasculitis • glomerulonephritis
Takayasu	"pulseless disease" • aorta / large arteries • Asian females
Kawasaki	mucocutaneous lymph node syndrome • coronary artery aneurysms • fever, conjunctivitis, maculopapular rash • Japanese children

Giant cell arteritis*: Early diagnosis is essential to prevent permanent loss of vision!*

1.34.) ANEURYSMS

	KEY FEATURES
atherosclerotic	• fusiform • abdominal aorta • hypertension
syphilitic	• saccular • ascending aorta • a/w aortic insufficiency
dissecting (not a "true" aneurysm)	• aorta (ascending or descending) • hypertension • Marfan syndrome
berry	• congenital • circle of Willis • a/w polycystic kidney disease (adult form)
micro	• cerebral : hypertension • retinal : diabetes

Abdominal aortic aneurysms are the most common due to atherosclerosis and hypertension. Rupture has a very high mortality! You must know which aneurysms are typical for each location.

1.35.) <u>HEART SOUNDS</u>

	OCCURS IN:	SOUNDS LIKE:
mitral valve prolapse	• young women • Marfan syndrome	• midsystolic click
mitral stenosis	• rheumatic heart disease • atrial fibrillation	• diastolic rumble
mitral regurgitation	• MI (papillary muscle) • acute rheumatic fever • endocarditis	• holosystolic murmur • transmitted *to axilla*
aortic stenosis	• congenital • degenerative calcification	• systolic murmur • transmitted *to carotid art.*
aortic regurgitation	• "water hammer" pulse	• diastolic murmur • "pistol shots" in femoral art.
patent ductus arteriosus	• kept open by PGE_2 , PGI_2	• continuous murmur ("machine like")

 Pulsus parvus et tardus*: "small and weak"* → *aortic stenosis*

1.36.) <u>CONGENITAL HEART DEFECTS</u>

R→L shunts (deoxygenated blood gets into the systemic circulation) are
more serious than L→R shunts (systemic blood gets into pulmonary circulation).

A) <u>TYPES</u>

ACYANOTIC (L→R)	CYANOTIC (R→L)	OBSTRUCTIVE

• VSD [1]
• ASD
  ostium primum
  ostium secundum
 	
• PDA
	• Fallot's tetralogy [1]
	• transposition of great vessels
	• persistent truncus arteriosus
	Eisenmenger : reversal of
	L→R shunt due to pulmonary
	hypertension
		• coarctation of aorta
		infants: preductal
		adults: postductal
		
		• pulmonary or aortic
		stenosis or atresia

[1] *most common cyanotic and acyanotic defects respectively*

B) <u>HEART DEFECTS ARE COMMON IN MANY SYNDROMES:</u>

	CARDIAC DEFECT PLUS:
fetal alcohol syndrome	• microcephaly • short, upturned nose, long philtrum
fetal hydantoin syndrome	• microcephaly • nail hypoplasia
isotretinoin (Vit. A)	• hydrocephalus • cleft palate
TORCH (intrauterine infection)	• microcephaly • auditory and visual defects
syphilis	• bullous skin lesions (palms, soles) • Hutchinson's teeth • saber shins

> **TORCH:** Toxoplasmosis, Rubella, CMV, Herpes

1.37.) ISCHEMIC HEART DISEASE

	SIGNS & TREATMENT
stable angina	• exercise • ST depression • relieved by rest ➢ *TX : nitroglycerin*
unstable angina	• at rest or crescendo like • often leads to MI ➢ *unresponsive to nitroglycerin*
Prinzmetal's angina	• at rest • ST elevated ➢ *TX : Ca^{2+} antagonists*

myocardial infarction	• during exercise or REM sleep
	• ST elevation
	• T inversion
	
	➢ *TX : nitroglycerin
	     morphine
	     lidocaine*

You should be able to make a diagnostic guess based on the clinical presentation. A suspect MI needs to be confirmed by ECG and enzymes:

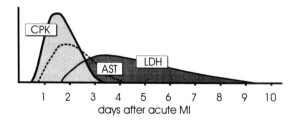

1.38.) <u>MYOCARDIAL INFARCTION</u>

Which complications occur early, which ones occur late?
How long does it take for an MI to heal?

TIME AFTER MI	GROSS CHANGE	MICROSCOPIC CHANGE
30 minutes	-	mitochondrial swelling
4-12 h	-	edema, hemorrhage
18-24 h	pallor	neutrophilic infiltrate
24-72 h	pallor	coagulation necrosis loss of nuclei heavy neutrophil. Infiltrate
3-7 days	central softening hyperemic borders	resorption of dead myofibers
10 days	max. soft and yellow hyperemic borders	granulation tissue
8 weeks	gray and firm scar	scar

<u>Complications</u>:

Arrhythmia: most common cause of death in first hours after MI
Myocardial rupture: highest risk 1~2 weeks after MI

most common

least common

arrhythmia
congestive heart failure
cardiogenic shock
muscle rupture

1.39.) HEART FAILURE

Left and right heart failure have very different signs and symptoms. It is important that you recognize the clinical presentation:

LEFT	RIGHT
CAUSES:	
• ischemic heart disease • arterial hypertension • valvular disease	• left sided heart failure • lung disease • primary pulmonary hypertension
CONSEQUENCES:	
• pulmonary congestion → dyspnea, orthopnea • renal hypoperfusion → salt retention	• increased venous pressure → edema → liver congestion ("nutmeg liver") → ascites

1.40.) ENDOCARDITIS

A) INFECTIVE

B) NON-INFECTIVE

ACUTE	SUBACUTE	MARANTIC	LIBMAN SACKS
• *Staph. aureus* • *Streptococci*	• *Strep. viridans* • *gram negative bacilli*	• a/w chronic illnesses	• SLE
• previously normal valves	• previously abnormal valves	• thrombotic (platelet and fibrin deposits)	• verrucous lesions on both sides of valve leaflets
• Janeway lesions	• Roth spots • Osler nodes		
• high fever, chills • hematuria	• low grade fever		

More common on the USMLE than in "real life":

Janeway lesions: non-tender, macular patches on palms and soles (septic emboli).
Roth spots: oval retinal hemorrhages with pale center.
Osler nodes: red, tender lesions on finger and toe pulps.

1.41.) <u>PERICARDITIS</u>

The space between the visceral and parietal pericardium normally contains ~20mL of clear fluid. The pathologist distinguishes 3 types of pericarditis based on the appearance of this fluid:

	KEY FEATURES
fibrinous	• transmural myocardial infarction, • Dressler syndrome • "bread and butter" appearance
serous	• viral infections (often Coxsackie) • uremia
suppurative	• bacterial infections • fungal infections • parasitic infections

<u>CLINICAL SIGNS:</u>
low-grade fever
pericardial friction rub: chest pain, aggravated by movement of trunk)
pulsus paradoxus: (nothing paradox about it) a normal inspiratory fall
in blood pressure that is exaggerated

Dressler syndrome*: Delayed pericarditis (2-10 weeks after infarction) due to auto-antibodies. Responds well to corticosteroids.*

1.42.) <u>RHEUMATIC FEVER</u>

Rheumatic fever occurs mostly in school age children
with untreated streptococcal pharyngitis.

ACUTE RHEUMATIC FEVER	RHEUMATIC HEART DISEASE
occurs 1-4 weeks after tonsillitis group A β-hemolytic streptococci	occurs many years after rheumatic fever often asymptomatic
common in children 5-15 years	fibrotic, deformed, calcified lines of closure on valve leaflets
<u>Major Jones Criteria</u> • polyarthritis • erythema • subcutaneous nodules • chorea • carditis	**mitral valve** > aortic valve

<u>Carditis of rheumatic fever</u>:
pericarditis → serous effusions
myocarditis → heart failure
endocarditis → valvular damage

ASCHOFF BODY:
- focal interstitial myocardial inflammation
- large myocytes (Anitschkow cells)
- multinucleated giant cells (Aschoff cells)

Most common clinical presentation is migratory
polyarthritis, lasting 2-3 weeks, accompanied by fever.

1.43.) OBSTRUCTIVE LUNG DISEASES

Reduced airflow either because airway resistance is high or because elastic recoil of lungs is low → **FRC and TLC are high.**

	KEY FEATURES
emphysema	• pink puffers , barrel chest • panacinar • (α1-antitrypsin deficiency, lower lobes) • centrilobular • (smoking, upper lobes)
chronic bronchitis	• blue bloaters • chronic irritation/ infections • hypertrophy of submucosal glands
asthma	• expiratory wheezing • extrinsic (triggered by allergens) • intrinsic (triggered by cold, exercise) [1] • aspirin induced
bronchiectasis	• result of chronic infections • Kartagener's : immotile cilia

[1] *intrinsic asthma is a common problem of ice skaters.*

COPD: usually coexisting:

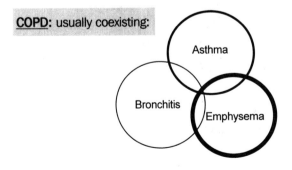

41

1.44.) <u>RESTRICTIVE LUNG DISEASES</u>

Elastic recoil of lungs is large → FRC , VC and TLC are low.

	KEY FEATURES
adult ARDS	• acute diffuse alveolar damage • (causes: sepsis, shock, pancreatitis, toxins)
neonatal ARDS	• insufficient lecithin synthesis by type 2 pneumocytes
pneumoconiosis	• coal : "tattooing", black sputum • anthracosis : carbon dust • asbestosis : fibrous silicates, dry cough • berylliosis : **Type IV hypersensitivity**
hypersensitivity pneumonitis	• acute : **(Type III)** fever, cough, dyspnea, leukocytosis • chronic : **(Type IV)** peribronchial granulomas • Farmer's lung, pigeon breeder's lung etc.
Goodpasture syndrome	• **(Type II)**, antibodies against basal membrane • hemoptysis, rapidly progressive glomerulonephritis
pulmonary hemosiderosis	• like Goodpasture's but without renal involvement
alveolar proteinosis	• overproduction of surfactant like material
eosinophilic pneumonia	• acute (Löffler's) : **Type I hypersensitivity** • chronic
diffuse idiopathic fibrosis	• interstitial pneumonitis and fibrosis • hyperplasia of type II pneumocytes
collagen vascular disorders	• scleroderma, SLE, Wegener's, RA etc.

Please review the immunological mechanisms of hypersensitivity (1.6) involved in restrictive lung diseases.

1.45.) PNEUMONIA

Sudden fever, cough, sputum and dyspnea are the signs of "classic pneumonia". It is a lobar pneumonia (affecting entire lobe of lung) caused by *Pneumococcus*.

	CAUSED BY
bronchopneumonia	• *Haemophilus* • *Pseudomonas*
lobar pneumonia ("classic")	• *Pneumococcus* • *Klebsiella*
atypical pneumonia [1]	• viral • *Mycoplasma*
Legionnaire's disease [2] (severe lobar pneumonia)	• *Legionella*

[1] *most frequent in young adults (college students)*

[2] *more frequent in elderly, via water reservoirs*
no person to person transmission

What is atypical about "atypical pneumonia"?
- more gradual onset
- dry, non productive cough
- minimal signs of pulmonary involvement during physical examination
- prominent extrapulmonary symptoms, myalgia etc.
- prominent chest x-ray ("looks worse than patient")

1.46.) LUNG TUMORS

A) NOT SMOKING RELATED:

benign	<ul><li>adenoma</li><li>leiomyoma</li><li>hamartoma</li></ul>
carcinoid	<ul><li>potentially malignant</li><li>carcinoid <u>syndrome</u> suggests widespread metastasis</li></ul>
adeno CA	<ul><li>peripheral, weakly related to smoking</li></ul>

B) SMOKING RELATED:

squamous CA	<ul><li>central, strong correlation with smoking</li><li>paraneoplastic: **PTH**-like peptide</li></ul>
small cell CA	<ul><li>central, hormone producing, aggressive</li><li>paraneoplastic: **ACTH, ADH**</li></ul>
large cell CA	<ul><li>peripheral, poorly differentiated adeno or squamous CA</li></ul>

<u>Clinical features:</u> (overall less than 5% 10-year survival)

- Pancoast tumor (apex of lung) → compressing cervical sympathetic chain
  → Horner's syndrome)

- Compression of recurrent laryngeal nerve → hoarseness
- Obstruction of superior vena cava → facial swelling

1.47.) GLOMERULONEPHRITIS - I

Clinically you must distinguish between nephritic and nephrotic syndrome:

NEPHRITIC SYNDROME	NEPHROTIC SYNDROME
• hematuria • RBC casts	• severe proteinuria • hypoalbuminemia • hyperlipidemia • edema
• post streptococcal GN	• adults: membranous GN • children: minimal change GN

The underlying pathology is established by renal biopsy and determines treatment and prognosis. But be aware that pathological changes and clinical manifestations often vary over time. You need to know which ones have a good and which have a poor prognosis:

diffuse proliferative GN	• poststreptococcal GN • good prognosis
mesangiocapillary GN (membranoproliferative GN)	• young adults, idiopathic • poor prognosis
focal-segmental GN	• aggressive variant of minimal change GN
Goodpasture's (anti-GBM antibodies)	• young males • pulmonary hemorrhage
Berger's (IgA nephropathy)	• very common, lasts 1-2 days • mild proteinuria, hematuria in children • follows respiratory infection

1.48.) GLOMERULONEPHRITIS - II

A) GOOD PROGNOSIS:

	CLINICAL FEATURES	PATHOLOGIC FEATURES
minimal change (lipoid nephrosis)	- most common nephrotic syndrome in children - insidious onset	- no immune complexes - **loss of foot processes**
diffuse proliferative	- nephritic/nephrotic - post streptococcal, SLE	- proliferation of mesangium and epithelium - **subepithelial deposits**

B) POOR PROGNOSIS:

	CLINICAL FEATURES	PATHOLOGIC FEATURES
membranous	- most common nephrotic syndrome in young adults - insidious onset	- thickening of GBM - **subepithelial deposits** of immune complexes - 85% unknown antigen
membrano-proliferative	- variable presentation	- GBM thickening plus proliferation of mesangium - **subendothelial or intra-membranous** deposits of immune complexes - "tram track" appearance
focal segmental	- related to minimal change?	- segmental sclerosis - usually IgM deposits (**IgA in Berger's**)
rapidly progressive	- aggressive variant of any other type	- **crescents** - oliguria, uremia

1.49.) <u>UROLITHIASIS</u>

Kidney stones form when the urine is supersaturated with salts. You need to know which salts precipitate in alkaline and which ones precipitate in acidic urine:

calcium	• 80% of cases • precipitates in **alkaline** urine ➢ *TX : thiazide* *potassium phosphate*
Mg - NH_3 – Phosphate "triple stones"	• (staghorn calculi) • urinary tract infections (*Proteus*) • precipitates in **alkaline** urine ➢ *TX : antibiotics* *acidification*
uric acid	• gout • leukemia • precipitates in **acidic** urine ➢ *TX : bicarbonate*
cystine	• congenital defect in dibasic • amino acid transporter • precipitates in **acidic** urine ➢ *TX : bicarbonate*

Renal colic: *excruciating, intermittent pain, radiating from flank area across abdomen to genital region.*

1.50.) VENEREAL DISEASES

	CAUSED BY:	CLINICAL FEATURES	TREATMENT
gonorrhea	*Neisseria gonorrhoeae*	purulent urethritis	ceftriaxone
trichomoniasis	*Trichomonas vaginalis*	men : asymptomatic or NGU female : vaginitis	metronidazole
non-gonococcal urethritis (NGU)	*Chlamydia trachomatis* [2]	urethritis, PID	doxycycline
lymphogranuloma venereum	*Chlamydia trachomatis* [2]	ulcer (**painless**) lymphadenopathy	doxycycline
granuloma inguinale	*C. donovani*	multiple ulcerating papules lymph nodes not involved [1]	tetracycline
chancroid	*Hemophilus ducreyi*	soft chancre (**painful**)	ceftriaxone
syphilis (I) **syphilis (II)** **syphilis (III)**	*Treponema pallidum*	hard chancre (**painless**) cond. lata (flat brown papules) gumma	penicillin G
condyloma acuminatum	HPV	"red warts"	cryotherapy
genital herpes	HSV2 or HSV1	recurrent vesicles (**painful**)	acyclovir

[1] *induration is of subcutaneous tissue*   [2] *different strains*

Yeast infection (*Candida*) is not sexually transmitted!

1.51.) TESTICULAR TUMORS

Patients present with a scrotal mass and you need to examine these carefully:
Testicular masses usually are malignant while extra-testicular ones often are benign.
Prognosis depends on tumor size and histology:

A) Germ Cell Tumors (common):

	KEY FEATURES
seminoma	• uniform polyhedral • radiosensitive, good prognosis
embryonal	• more aggressive • hemorrhage, necrosis
choriocarcinoma	• highly malignant • gynecomastia
yolk sac	• most common in children • serum AFP ↑ • very aggressive
teratoma	• contains multiple tissue types • often malignant!

B) Non Germ Cell Tumors (rare):

Leydig cell	• androgens, estrogens, corticosteroids • usually benign
Sertoli cell	• little or no hormone production
lymphoma	• most common in elderly

1.52.) <u>OVARIAN TUMORS</u>

A) <u>Surface Endothelium</u> (most common):

	KEY FEATURES
<u>serous</u>	• cysts, ciliated epithelium
<u>mucinous</u>	• cysts, non ciliated epithelium
<u>endometrioid</u>	• glandular tissue
<u>clear cell</u>	• rare, malignant
Brenner	• rare, benign • nests of <u>transitional</u> epithelium in stroma

B) <u>Germ Cell Tumors</u> (less common):

<u>teratoma</u>	• usually mature (benign) [1]
<u>dysgerminoma</u>	• like seminoma, radiosensitive
<u>endodermal sinus tumor</u>	• like yolk sac tumor, AFP ↑
choriocarcinoma	• produces HCG

[1] *also called dermoid cyst*

C) <u>SEX CORD</u> Stroma Cell Tumors (rare):

<u>granulosa-theca</u>	• estrogens and androgens
<u>Sertoli-Leydig</u>	• androgens → masculinization
fibroma	• Meig's syndrome → ascites

Compare ovarian tumors side by side with testicular tumors.
Which correspond to which?

1.53.) ENDOMETRIUM

Proliferation of endometrial glands due to estrogen stimulation results in:

POLYPS	HYPERPLASIA	CARCINOMA
• excessive bleeding • rarely malignant transformation	• excessive bleeding • premalignant	• usually adenocarcinoma • may be asymptomatic or present with bleeding
		risk factors age >40 years early menarche late menopause nulliparity obesity

1.54.) PLACENTA

HYDATIDIFORM MOLE (80% benign)	CHORIOCARCINOMA (malignant)

• older pregnant woman
• uterus larger than expected
• grape-like cystic material
 	
• HCG elevated
	• derived from : hydatidiform mole (50%)
	  pregnancy (25%)
	  abortion (25%)
	
	• HCG elevated

 Moles are due to fertilization of ovum by multiple sperms:

Complete hydatidiform mole:
o   no embryo or placenta
o   46,XX of exclusively paternal origin

Partial hydatidiform mole:
o   embryo and placenta are present
o   triploid or tetraploid karyotype

1.55.) <u>BREAST</u>

Most breast masses are benign. Please compare carefully:

FIBROCYSTIC CHANGE	BREAST CANCER
<ul><li>often bilateral</li><li>multiple nodules</li><li>menstrual variation</li><li>may regress during pregnancy</li></ul>	<ul><li>often unilateral</li><li>single mass</li><li>no cyclic variations</li></ul>

<u>BENIGN TUMORS</u>

fibroadenoma	• single, movable nodule
cystosarcoma phyllodes	• rapidly growing, may become huge
intraductal papilloma	• nipple discharge (bloody or serous) • nipple retraction

<u>MALIGNANT TUMORS</u>

ductal carcinoma	• most common
lobular carcinoma	• if receptor positive → better prognosis
Paget's disease of nipple	• older woman • poor prognosis

> **<u>Risk factors for breast cancer:</u>**
> same as for endometrial cancer (1.53)

5% of women with breast cancer carry BRCA1 or BRCA2 gene. Women without positive family history probably do not carry these genes and screening for BRCA1 or BRCA2 is not recommended.

1.56.) <u>MOUTH</u>

Some diseases cause characteristic changes of the lips, gums or tongue:

bleeding gums	Vit. C deficiency
glossitis, cheilosis	Vit. B2 deficiency
smooth beefy red tongue	Vit. B12 deficiency
strawberry tongue	scarlet fever
Koplik's spots (white dots on red background)	measles
thrush (white, removable)	Candida albicans

1.57.) <u>ESOPHAGEAL DIVERTICULA</u>

PULSION DIVERTICULA (Zenker's)	TRACTION DIVERTICULA
• "false" (mucosa only)	• "true" (all layers)
• at junction of pharynx/esophagus	• mid part of esophagus
• dysphagia, regurgitation	• asymptomatic

Compare the anatomic features of the two types of diverticula and review the layers of the gastrointestinal tube: mucosa → lamina propria → muscularis mucosa → submucosa → circular muscle layer → longitudinal muscle layer.

1.58.) GASTRITIS

"Gastritis" is 4 different, unrelated diseases:

ACUTE EROSIVE	CHRONIC TYPE A	CHRONIC TYPE B	MÉNÉTRIER'S
focal damage • alcohol • NSAIDs • stress	fundal gastritis • autoimmune • pernicious anemia • achlorhydria	antral gastritis • *H. pylori*	thickened mucosa

 Patients on intensive care often develop acute erosive gastritis. You may want to give prophylactic anti-histamine (H_2).

H. pylori is associated with:
- chronic gastritis type B
- gastric and duodenal peptic ulcers
- carcinoma of stomach

1.59.) GASTROENTERITIS

TOXIN INGESTION	BACTERIA	NON-BACTERIAL
Staph. aureus *Cl. botulinum*	**toxigenic** *Campylobacter* [1] *E. coli* *Salmonella* **invasive** *Shigella*	Rotavirus (children) Parvovirus (adults) Candida Entameba histolytica Giardia lamblia

[1] *most common in US !*

1.60.) POLYPOSIS OF COLON

Step by Step:

Absence of APC (a tumor suppressor gene) causes familial adenomatous polyposis. If the adenoma cells develop an additional mutation of the normal gene on the other allele, they will become cancerous!

		POLYPS PLUS:	CANCER RISK:
familial adenomatous polyposis	autosomal dominant	(none)	almost 100%
Gardner's	autosomal dominant	+ skin and bone tumors	almost 100%
Turcot's	autosomal recessive	+ brain tumors	high
Peutz-Jeghers	autosomal dominant	+ melanin pigmentation of lips, palms and soles	very low

Follow-up and genetic counseling:

- Patient's off-spring has 50% risk of disease.
- Screen annually until age 35 (flexible sigmoidoscopy)
- If polyps develop → need to remove colon.

1.61.) INFLAMMATORY BOWEL DISEASE

A favorite on the USMLE. You must memorize the differences:

CROHN'S DISEASE	ULCERATIVE COLITIS
• rectum often spared • ileum often involved	• begins at rectum and progresses • towards ileocecal junction
• skip lesions • transmural	• continuous • mucosa / submucosa only
• granulomas • strictures and fissures	• crypt abscesses • pseudopolyps
• more pain, less bleeding	• more bleeding, less pain
	complications: - increased risk of colon carcinoma - toxic megacolon

1.62.) MALABSORPTION

celiac sprue	• toxic/allergic reaction against gluten • flat mucosal surface • avoid wheat • rice and corn are O.K.
tropical sprue	• cause unknown
Whipple's disease	• malabsorption + anemia + arthritis • *Tropheryma whippelii* • PAS positive macrophages found in mucosa ➢ *TX : penicillin or tetracycline*

Symptoms are due to (1.) osmotically active substances remaining in the GI tract (diarrhea, bloating) and (2.) nutritional deficiencies (weight loss, glossitis, megaloblastic anemia).

1.63.) CHOLELITHIASIS

Cholesterol is insoluble in water and must be incorporated in salt-phospholipid micelles in the bile. Supersaturation results in crystal formation and stones.

STONE TYPES:

CHOLESTEROL	MIXED	PIGMENT (BILIRUBIN)
• radiolucent [1] • often a single stone • Westerners • fat, female, forty, fertile	• most common • 15% radiopaque	• radiolucent [1] • a/w hemolytic anemia • Asians

[1] *not detectable on plain radiograph*

Porcelain Gallbladder: - calcium deposits in wall
                                   - high risk of malignancy

Strawberry Gallbladder: - asymptomatic lipid deposits
                                   - not related to cholelithiasis
                                   - no cancer risk

Charcot's triad (= cholangitis):
1. acute onset fever, sepsis
2. RUQ pain
3. jaundice

1.64.) CARCINOMA

Curiously, gallbladder and bile duct carcinomas are quite different:

GALLBLADDER CA	BILE DUCT CA
• female • cholelithiasis • porcelain gallbladder	• male • chronic infections • liver fluke (*Clonorchis sinensis*)

1.65.) <u>JAUNDICE</u>

occurs when serum bilirubin > 2 mg/dl
direct   = conjugated   = water soluble
indirect = unconjugated = insoluble (bound to albumin)

	DUE TO:	SERUM BILIRUBIN
prehepatic	hemolysis	unconjugated
hepatic	hepatitis	conjugated and unconjugated
posthepatic	cholestasis	conjugated

<u>CONGENITAL CAUSES OF JAUNDICE</u> :

Gilbert	auto-dominant	impaired uptake (mild)
Crigler-Najjar	auto-dominant or auto-recessive	impaired uptake (very severe)
Rotor	auto-recessive	impaired hepatocellular secretion

Physiologic jaundice of the newborn:
2-3 days after birth
lasts less than 1 week
more severe in prematures
(immature liver enzymes abd immature blood-brain barrier)

1.66.) <u>HEPATITIS</u>

The clinical presentation varies from minor flu-like illness to fulminant, fatal liver failure. Histopathology is similar, regardless of the specific virus. You should know the serum markers (for diagnosis) and routes of transmission (for prevention):

A	RNA	• viruses in feces • acute : IgM • late : IgG	• **fecal/oral** • 2-6 weeks [2] • 0% chronic
B	DNA	• HBs-Ag , earliest marker [1] • HBe-Ag, infective state	• **parenteral** • 2-6 months [2] • 10% chronic
C	RNA	• antibody ELISA	• **parenteral** • 1-2 months [2] • 50% chronic
Delta	RNA	• incomplete RNA • requires Hep B virus for replication	• **parenteral**
E	RNA		• **fecal oral** • SE Asia • often fulminant in pregnant woman

[1] *also indicates carrier state*   [2] *incubation times*

<u>CHRONIC HEPATITIS</u> (> 6 months):
chronic persistent hepatitis
• inflammation limited to portal triad

chronic active hepatitis
• inflammation beyond portal triad (piece meal necrosis)

1.67.) HEPATITIS B SEROLOGY

These markers are important for diagnosis and follow-up:

HBeAg	• appears after HBsAg • disappears before HBsAg • indicates infectivity!
HBsAg	• appears before onset of symptoms • persists for 3-4 months • if > 6 months: chronic carrier state
anti-HBsAg	• appears a few weeks after HBsAg has disappeared • indicates recovery and immunity
anti HBcAg	• only marker present during "window period"

*"**Window period**": time after HBsAg disappears but before anti-HBsAg appears in patient's serum.*

1.68.) TOXIC HEPATITIS

Many drugs can cause hepatitis in a predictable, dose-depend manner. A few drugs elicit a severe, idiosyncratic (dose-independent) hepatitis in susceptible patients:

PREDICTABLE	IDIOSYNCRATIC
➢ acetaminophen ➢ amanita ➢ carbon tetrachloride ➢ methotrexate	➢ halothane ➢ isoniazid ➢ methyl-DOPA

1.69.) CIRRHOSIS

A) Most common types of cirrhosis:

ALCOHOL (60%)	TOXINS, VIRAL (30%)	BILIARY (10%)
early: micronodular **late** : macronodular	macronodular	micronodular
Mallory bodies [1] in <u>acute</u> hepatitis !		autoimmune disease anti-mitochondrial antibodies

[1] *swollen hepatocytes that contain cytoplasmic inclusions of a fibrillar protein. NOT specific for alcohol hepatitis!*

B) Rare types of cirrhosis:

HEMOCHROMATOSIS: - accumulation of hemosiderin
triad of (1.) cirrhosis, (2.) diabetes mellitus and (3.) skin pigmentation

WILSON'S DISEASE: - accumulation of copper
                      - decreased serum ceruloplasmin

1.70.) LIVER CARCINOMA

METASTATIC	HEPATOCELLULAR	CHOLANGIOCARCINOMA
most common	90% of <u>primary</u> ones	10% of <u>primary</u> ones
• from breast • from lung • from colon	HBV and HCV aflatoxin AFP ↑	more common in Asia (liver fluke)

1.71.) ARTHRITIS

You should be able to distinguish the clinical presentation of osteoarthritis and rheumatoid arthritis:

OSTEOARTHRITIS	RHEUMATOID ARTHRITIS (RA)
• women > men	• women 20~50 years
• loss of cartilage • narrowing of joint space • increased density of subchondral bone • osteophyte formation	• synovial membrane proliferation (pannus) • erosions of cartilage and subchondral bone
• knees, hips, spine • distal interphalangeal joints	• starts in small joints • proximal interphalangeal joints • metacarpophalangeal joints
• joint stiffness after inactivity (e.g. sitting in chair) • Heberden's nodes	• morning stiffness • soft tissue swelling • rheumatoid nodules (skin, valves..) • rheumatoid factor: anti IgG

Heberden's nodes are osteophytes at the distal interphalangeal joints.

STILL'S DISEASE:
juvenile RA, acute febrile, no rheumatoid factors

PSORIATIC ARTHRITIS:
like RA, but absence of rheumatoid factors

FELTY'S SYNDROME:
polyarticular RA, splenomegaly, leukopenia, leg ulcers

1.72.) <u>BONES</u>

A) <u>CONGENITAL</u>:

	KEY FEATURES
osteogenesis imperfecta	• disorder of collagen synthesis • fractures • blue, thin sclera
osteopetrosis	• increased density • brittle bones • facial distortion due to bone overgrowth
achondroplasia	• autosomal dominant • defective cartilage synthesis • decreased epiphyseal formation • short limbs, normal size head and trunk

B) <u>ACQUIRED</u>:
Diagnosis is made by X-ray and lab tests:

OSTEOPOROSIS	OSTEOMALACIA	PAGET'S
- thinned cortical bone - enlarged medullary cavity	- diffuse radiolucency	- bones enlarged and radiolucent
- normal Ca and phosphate - normal alk. phosphatase	- low Ca, low phosphate - high alk. phosphatase	- extremely high alkaline phosphatase
- decreased bone mass - estrogen deficiency - immobilization - Cushing's syndrome	- impaired mineralization - lack of Vit. D - chronic renal insufficiency	- excessive bone resorption with replacement

1.73.) CARTILAGE

Three types of cartilage differ by the composition of their extracellular matrix:

hyaline cartilage	type II collagen o joints o developing bones o joints o trachea/larynx o nose
elastic cartilage	elastin o ear
fibrocartilage	type I collagen o intervertebral disks o menisci

A) BENIGN TUMORS:

	KEY FEATURES
osteochondroma	• developmental defect • exostosis at metaphyseal projections
enchondroma	• may develop into chondrosarcoma • cartilage within bone
chondroblastoma	• benign • femur, tibia, humerus epiphysis

B) MALIGNANT TUMORS:

	KEY FEATURES
chondrosarcoma	• malignant • spine, pelvic bones • slower growing than osteosarcoma

1.74.) BONE TUMORS

Diagnosis can often be made from location and typical X-ray appearance and should be considered together with the histopathology. You should know which tumors are benign and which are malignant:

A) BENIGN TUMORS:

	KEY FEATURES
osteoma	• benign • skull
osteoid osteoma	• benign, painful • tibia or femur (diaphysis)
osteoblastoma	• like osteoid osteoma • larger but painless • may be malignant

B) MALIGNANT TUMORS:

	KEY FEATURES
osteosarcoma	• highly malignant • metaphysis of long bone (knee) • Codman's triangle
Ewing's sarcoma	• very aggressive • young males • pelvis, long bones • within marrow cavity • "onion skin" appearance

1.75.) <u>MUSCULAR DYSTROPHIES</u>

Dystrophies cause progressive weakness of select muscle groups.
Unfortunately, the most severe form is also the most common one:

	KEY FEATURES
Duchenne	X linked **absent dystrophin protein** • most severe • pelvic girdle weakness • pseudohypertrophy of calves
Becker	X linked **abnormal dystrophin protein** • less severe than Duchenne • may walk until age 20-25
limb girdle	**autosomal recessive** • late onset
facioscapulohumeral	**autosomal dominant** • late onset
myotonic	**autosomal dominant** • late onset • limb involvement is distal • inability to voluntarily relax muscle

Gower's sign: *When trying to stand up the child uses its hands to climb up himself.*

Clinical features (Duchenne):
• presents in boys age 3-7
• proximal muscle weakness → waddling gait
• pseudohypertrophy: fatty and fibrous infiltration of calve muscle
• increased serum CPK

1.76.) BRAIN TUMORS

Try to get a "feel" for which ones are relatively benign and which ones are highly malignant:

		KEY FEATURES
Neural Tube	astrocytoma	• slow growing, M > F
	glioblastoma	• always fatal, M > F
	medulloblastoma	• children, M > F
	oligodendroblastoma	• rare, M = F slow growing, seizures
Neural Crest	meningioma	• from arachnoid, benign, F > M "whorling pattern" psammoma bodies
	Schwannoma	• acoustic neurinoma, F > M a/w von Recklinghausen's
	neurofibroma	• fibroblasts and Schwann cells, benign usually von Recklinghausen's
Ectoderm	craniopharyngioma	• most common supratentorial tumor in children, compresses optic nerve
	pituitary adenoma	• 60% prolactin (chromophobe) • 10% growth hormone (eosinophil) • 10% ACTH (basophil)
Mesoderm	lymphoma	• B cells, periventricular
	lipoma	• "egg shell" appearance
	hemangioblastoma	

1.77.) CNS DEGENERATION

Alzheimer's is the most common degenerative disease of the CNS. It's pathological features are (1.) diffuse cortical atrophy, (2.) senile plaques (amyloid protein), and (3.) neurofibrillary tangles (cytoplasmic deposit of tau protein).
Please compare with the less common degenerative diseases of the CNS:

	KEY FEATURES
Pick's	• lobar atrophy • mainly frontal and temporal
Parkinson's	• bradykinesia, rigidity, resting tremor • dopamine depletion (caudate, putamen) • **Lewy bodies** (spherical inclusions in melanin-depleted neurons of the substantia nigra)
ALS	• rapidly progressive • degeneration of corticospinal tract (UMN) • degeneration of α-motoneurons (LMN)
Huntington's	• chorea, athetoid movements • atrophy of caudate, putamen and frontal cortex
Friedreich's ataxia	• autosomal recessive • pes cavus • loss of proprioception • tremors, Babinski reflex • spinal cord atrophy • (spinocerebellar, corticospinal, post. columns)

Upper motor neuron lesions: spasticity, increased tendon reflexes
Lower motor neuron lesions: paralysis, fasciculations, absent tendon reflexes

1.78.) <u>DEMYELINATING DISEASES</u>

Myelin sheaths are composed of lipoproteins and formed by the oligodendroglia (CNS) or Schwann cells (peripherally). Congenital metabolic disorders affect the developing myelination and results in severe neurological deficits.

Demyelination occurring in later life can be repaired by the glia. This explains the frequent exacerbations and remissions in MS.

	KEY FEATURES
multiple sclerosis	• onset at age 20-40 • a/w cool, temperate climate • oligoclonal bands
Devic's	• like MS, but **limited** to spinal chord and optical nerve
Guillain-Barré	• peripheral nerves (mainly motor) • autoimmune, often following viral infection
adrenoleukodystrophy	• X linked • accumulation of long chain cholesterols • blindness, ataxia • latent adrenal insufficiency
Schilder's	• focal demyelination in brain • children • visual, auditory, motor defects • variant of adrenoleukodystrophy

<u>Oligoclonal bands (CSF electrophoresis):</u>
- o Multiple monoclonal gamma globulins.
- o Characteristic, but not entirely specific for MS.

1.79.) <u>PITUITARY HYPERFUNCTION</u>

<u>ANTERIOR PITUITARY:</u>

eosinophile cells	prolactin	**male** : decreased libido, impotence **female** : galactorrhea, amenorrhea, infertility
	GH	**prepubertal** : giantism **adults** : acromegaly
basophile cells	ACTH	**Cushing's disease** is the most common cause of Cushing's syndrome (except iatrogenic)

Classification according to staining properties is outdated since there is only an approximate relationship between hormones and cell staining.

While prolactin is mainly produced by eosinophil cells, prolactinomas are usually **chromophobe** !

1.80.) <u>PITUITARY HYPOFUNCTION</u>

Sheehan's syndrome (ischemic necrosis, often postpartum)	<u>panhypopituitarism:</u> • hypothyroidism • hypoadrenalism • hypogonadism
dwarfism	a) growth hormone deficiency b) lack of receptors (e.g. in pygmies)
eunuchoid hypogonadism, primary amenorrhea	gonadotropin deficiency (common!)

1.81.) ADRENAL ADENOMAS/CARCINOMAS

The adrenal gland has 2 distinct components: The cortex producing steroids and the medulla, derived from the neuro crest, producing epinephrine and norepinephrine.

cortex : adenoma	most adenomas do <u>not</u> produce steroids **Conn:** mineralocorticoids ↑ **Cushing:** glucocorticoids ↑ **Virilization:** androgens ↑
cortex : carcinoma	much rarer than adenomas, but if they occur they usually produce hormones!
medulla : pheochromocytoma	**10%** extra-adrenal **10%** bilateral **10%** malignant
neuroblastoma	common tumor in children < 5 years from medulla or sympathetic chain ganglia

CONN:
- hypernatremia → hypervolemia → high blood pressure
- potassium loss → muscle weakness

CUSHING:
- "moon face", "buffalo hump"
- truncal obesity
- skin striae
- osteoporosis
- low glucose tolerance

Mineral corticoids	zona Glomerulosa
Glucocorticoids	zona Fasciculata
Androgens	zona Reticularis

"The deeper you go the sweeter it gets!"

1.82.) THYROID

Like the adrenals, the thyroid gland also has 2 distinct components: **(1.)** follicle cells produce T4 and T3, **(2.)** parafollicular C-cells make calcitonin. T3 is derived by removal of iodine from T4 in the blood and is much more potent!

		KEY FEATURES
hyperthyroidism :	**Graves'** (diffuse toxic goiter)	• lymphocytes • small follicles • little colloid
	Plummer's (nodular toxic goiter)	• hyperplasia, hypertrophy • colloid accumulation
hypothyroidism :	**diffuse simple goiter** (iodine deficiency)	• hyperplasia, hypertrophy
	Hashimoto's	• lymphocytes, plasma cells • atrophic follicles • little colloid
	Riedel's	• fibrous replacement
euthyroid :	**De Quervain's**	• viral • leakage of colloid • granulomas

"Sick euthyroid" syndrome:
- Many patients with severe illness, trauma or stress have low T3 and low T4, but clinically no signs of hypothyroidism.
- TSH is also normal in these cases.

1.83.) THYROID TUMORS

		KEY FEATURES
benign :	follicular adenoma	• very common • most are cold nodules
malignant :	papillary CA	• younger patients • a/w radiation exposure • Psammoma bodies
	follicular CA	• adenomatous pattern
	anaplastic CA	• undifferentiated • poor prognosis
	medullary CA	• parafollicular (C cells)

 Medullary CA of the thyroid is often a/w MEN type II.

- **Papillary carcinoma** is more **common** than follicular carcinoma.
- **Follicular carcinoma** is more **aggressive** than papillary carcinoma.

1.84.) PARATHYROIDS

Derived from the 3rd and 4th pharyngeal pouches, these glands produce PTH. PTH acts on bone osteoclasts and mobilizes calcium.

	KEY FEATURES
hyperparathyroidism	<u>primary</u> adenoma *** <u>secondary</u> chronic renal failure Vit. D deficiency
hypoparathyroidism	• thyroidectomy *** • DiGeorge's syndrome ➢ PTH low ➢ Ca^{2+} low
pseudohypo...	• receptor defect • short stature • short metacarpal bones ➢ PTH elevated ➢ Ca^{2+} low
pseudopseudohypo...	• same physical appearance as in pseudohypoparathyroidism ➢ PTH normal ➢ Ca^{2+} levels normal

*** *most common causes, respectively*

<u>Renal osteodystrophy:</u>
chronic renal failure→ decreased phosphate excretion
→ phosphate binds ionized calcium in serum
→ hypocalcemia
→ increased PTH
→ bone demineralization

TX: Aluminum may be used to bind phosphate.

1.85.) DIABETES MELLITUS

Most common endocrine disease → serious morbidity

A) PRIMARY DIABETES:

IDDM (Type I)	NIDDM (Type II)	MODY
• not so common	• very common	• rare
• juvenile onset • prone to ketoacidosis	• adult onset • not prone to ketoacidosis	• juvenile onset
• viral etiology?	• inadequate insulin secretion • obesity, insulin resistance	• glucokinase defect (glucose sensor)
• weak genetic predisposition [1] (HLA DR 3, DR4)	• strong genetic predisposition [2]	
• auto-immune (islet cell antibodies)	• hyalinization of islets	
• decreased number of β-cells		

[1] *<50% concordance*   [2] *100% concordance in monozygotic twins*

B) SECONDARY DIABETES:

hemochromatosis	chronic pancreatitis, pancreas carcinoma
"bronze diabetes"	→ islet cell destruction

Gestational diabetes: 1-3% of women develop diabetes during pregnancy. This induces excessive fetal insulin secretion and increases the risk of birth trauma (increased fetal weight due to the metabolic effects of insulin). Usually glucose tolerance returns to normal after delivery, but 30% of women with gestational diabetes develop overt diabetes mellitus within 5 years.

1.86.) <u>MULTIPLE ENDOCRINE NEOPLASIA</u>

MEN is inherited autosomal dominant with variable penetrance. MEN Type 1 is due to loss of a tumor suppressor gene. Neoplasia arises when the second, healthy allele of this gene mutates.

MEN Type 1	MEN Type 2A	MEN Type 2B
• adrenal <u>cortex</u> • pituitary • parathyroid • pancreas (gastrinoma)	• adrenal <u>medulla</u> • thyroid medulla • parathyroid	• adrenal <u>medulla</u> • thyroid medulla • mucosal neuromas • marfanoid features
"pity-para-pan"	"para-medullary-medulla"	

CLINICAL PRESENTATIONS:

MEN 1:   (90%) primary hyperparathyroidism → hypercalcemia
             (70%) gastrin → Zollinger-Ellison syndrome → peptic ulcers
             (60%) pituitary tumors → visual disturbances
                     (sometimes produce GH → acromegaly)

MEN 2A: (100%) medullary carcinoma of thyroid (bilateral)
                    → early diagnosis is essential!
             (50%) benign pheochromocytoma (bilateral)
                    → hypertensive crisis (headache, sweating, palpitations)
             (20%) primary hyperparathyroidism → hypercalcemia

Hypercalcemia is either asymptomatic or may produce kidney stones.

1.87.) SKIN TUMORS

Skin cancer is the most common cancer in the US and directly related to sun-exposure. 80% of these are basal cell carcinomas with very low metastatic potential.

A) BENIGN:

	KEY FEATURES
seborrheic keratosis	• brownish/gray, scaly, greasy
keratoacanthoma	• rapidly growing pink papula • looks like squamous cell carcinoma but is benign
actinic keratosis	• crusty red papule, premalignant

B) MALIGNANT:

	KEY FEATURES
basal cell carcinoma	• pearly, gray papule
squamous cell carcinoma	• erythematous, scaly or oozing ulcer • Bowen's disease: squamous CA in situ
melanoma	• brown, black, red, white, purple, irregular borders • lentigo maligna: grows horizontally • nodular melanoma: grows vertically

---

The "ABC" of melanoma:
A - asymmetric lesion
B - borders irregular
C - color variations

1.88.) <u>OTHER SKIN DISEASES</u>

Spend a day with a dermatology atlas and learn to recognize these:

	KEY FEATURES
pemphigus	• vesicles on mucosa • auto antibodies against intercellular junctions of keratinocytes
pemphigoid	• like pemphigus, but larger bullae on abdomen and groin
impetigo	• honey colored crust, superficial skin infection • *Staphylococcus* or β-hemolytic *Streptococci*
pityriasis	• (viral cause?) • herald patch → spreads along flexural lines
rosacea	• large, red nose

	KEY FEATURES
xanthoma	• hyperlipidemia, foamy histocytes
capillary hemangioma	• "salmon patches" and stork bites *spontaneously regresses* • "strawberry hemangiomas" *initially grows, later regresses*
cavernous hemangioma	• "port-wine stain", a/w Sturge-Weber *does not resolve spontaneously*
café-au-lait spots	• a/w von neurofibromatosis
vitiligo	• irregular depigmentation

79

1.89.) TOXINS

	PATHOLOGY
cadmium	"honeycomb" pneumonitis
cobalt	cardiomyopathy
chromium	lung cancer
lead	inhibits heme synthesis renal tubular acidosis
mercury	neurotoxic (Minamata !) proximal tubular necrosis
arsenic	lung cancer
asbestos	mesothelioma
aromatic amines	bladder cancer
benzene	leukemia
vinyl chloride	liver angiosarcoma
α-amanitin	fulminant hepatitis
CO	forms carboxyhemoglobin[1]
cyanide	inhibits mitochondrial cytochromes → loss of O_2 utilization

[1] *do not confuse with methemoglobin, which contains oxidized Fe^{3+}*

Hot-Pics

Be able to recognize the following pictures:

MICROSCOPIC:

- **Amyloid:** birefringence
- **Red blood cells:** microcytic hypochrome versus macrocytic megaloblastic
  target cells
  sickle cells
- **White blood cells:** ALL versus AML
- **Reed-Sternberg cell** (Hodgkin's disease)
- **Barrett's esophagus:** metaplasia
- **Granulomas:** caseating (TBC) versus non-caseating (foreign body)
- **Lung:** acid fast bacilli
  Aspergillus,
  Pneumocystis carinii (silver stain)
- **Lung:** oat cell carcinoma
- **Breast:** normal versus fibroadenoma versus cancer
- **Kaposi sarcoma**
- **Teratoma:** skin, teeth, neural tissue etc.
- **Giant cell arteritis**
- **Bacterial pneumonia**
- **Kidneys:** hypertensive change
- **Kidney immunofluorescence**: linear pattern (Goodpasture's syndrome)
  granular pattern (membranous GN)
  mesangial pattern (IgA nephropathy)
- **Colon:** adenomatous polyp versus adenocarcinoma
- **Liver:** hepatitis, fatty degeneration
- **Ovary:** Krukenberg tumor (signet ring cells)
- **Cervix:** carcinoma in situ
- **Pap smear:** dysplastic cell versus glycogen rich normal cells
- **CNS:** Alzheimer's disease: neurofibrillary tangles, plaques
  Parkinson's disease: depigmentation of substantia nigra

MACROSCOPIC:

- **Cardiac hypertrophy:** eccentric versus concentric hypertrophy
- **Breast carcinoma:** (mammography)
- **Lung:** Ghon complex (X-ray)
- **Gall-bladder:** stone types
- **Hydatidiform mole**
- **Pituitary adenoma** (X-ray of sella turcica)
- **Brain:** atrophy of cortex
       atrophy of caudate nucleus

MICROBIOLOGY

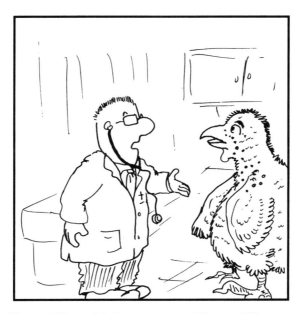

"It could be chicken pox, but then all these
viruses look similar."

Part A : General Microbiology

Stains take advantage of special properties in the cell walls from different organisms. The most famous is Gram, separating bacteria roughly into 3 classes :
1. **Gram+**: Bacteria that are rich in peptidoglycan retain violet dye.
2. **Gram -** : Bacteria that are poor in peptidoglycan but counterstain with red dye.
3. Bacteria that do not stain with either dye, requiring "special stains".

2.1.) STAINS

	USED FOR:
Ziehl Neelsen	stains acid fast bacteria red
India ink	cryptococcus
Giemsa	blood smears
PAS	glycogen, mucopolysaccharides
Prussian blue	iron
Congo red	amyloid
osmic acid	for electron microscopy

GRAM STAIN:
1. Crystal violet dye (plus iodine) stains all bacterial cell walls.
2. Alcohol extracts blue dye from lipid-rich, thin-walled gram-negative bacteria.
3. Red dye counterstains decolorized gram-negative bacteria.
4. Gram-positive bacteria remain blue.

2.2.) <u>NORMAL FLORA</u>

Normal flora are microorganisms that are found in particular sites in healthy people. Often, they have a symbiotic relationship with the host. (1.) They stimulate the immune system of newborns. (2.) They interfere with colonization by pathogenic strains.

	USUAL FLORA	POTENTIAL PATHOGENS
skin	*Staph. epidermidis*	*Staph. aureus*
nasopharynx	*Strep. viridans* anaerobes	*Strep. pneumoniae* *N. meningitides* *H. influenzae*
mouth	*Strep. viridans*	*Candida albicans*
colon	*E. coli*	*Bacteroides fragilis* enterococci
vagina	*Lactobacillus* *Streptococci*	*Candida albicans*

<u>Clinical examples</u>:
- Risk of endocarditis after dental procedures (*Strep. viridans*).
- Pseudomembranous colitis following administration of broad-spectrum antibiotics (*Cl. difficile* usually suppressed by endogenous flora)

2.3.) <u>CELL WALLS</u>

all bacteria (except mycoplasma)	**inner layer of cell wall: peptidoglycans** • thick in gram-positives • thin in gram-negatives
gram-positive	**outer layer of cell wall:** teichoic acid
gram-negative	**outer layer of cell wall:** lipopolysaccharides (=endotoxins) • outer cell membrane (lipid bilayer) [1] • porins
mycobacteria	• mycolic acid in cell wall (resists decoloration of gram-stain)
mycoplasma	• has no cell wall • only bacterium whose membrane contains cholesterol!
spores	• dipicolinic acid (keratin coat) → resistance to heat, dehydration and chemicals

[1] *the space between outer membrane and cell membrane contains*
β-lactamase (degrades penicillins).

<u>CELL CAPSULE:</u>
• composed of polysaccharides
• determines virulence
• capsular antigens determine species
• vaccines are made against capsular antigens

2.4.) <u>TOXINS</u>

Exotoxins are made by Gram+ and Gram- bacteria, are proteins and can be neutralized by antibodies (=antitoxins). Endotoxins are lipopolysaccharides from Gram- bacteria and are poorly antigenic.

ENDOTOXINS	<ul><li>lipopolysaccharides</li><li>non-specific</li><li>TNF, IL-1 → fever, shock</li><li>poor antigen</li><li>heat **stable**</li></ul>
EXOTOXINS	<ul><li>polypeptides</li><li>specific</li><li>toxoids used as vaccine</li><li>usually **heat labile**</li></ul>
tetanus toxin	• blocks release of glycine → muscle spasms
botulinum toxin	• blocks release of ACh → muscle paralysis
diphtheria toxin	• inhibits protein synthesis (ADP-ribosylation of EF-2)
alpha toxin	*Staph. aureus* • hemolysis, necrosis, cell death
toxic shock syndrome toxin	*Staph. aureus* • induces cytokines → anaphylactic shock
cholera toxin	• stimulates adenylate cyclase (activates G_s)
pertussis toxin	• stimulates adenylate cyclase (inhibits G_i)
enterotoxin	*E. coli* • **heat labile:** stimulates adenylate cyclase • **heat stable:** stimulates guanylate cyclase

2.5.) O₂-REQUIREMENTS

Aerobes require O_2 and cannot ferment.
Obligate anaerobes ferment and are killed by O_2.
Microaerophilics grow best at low O_2 but also can grow without O_2.

obligate aerobe	• M. tuberculosis • Pseudomonas aeruginosa • Nocardia
microaerophilic	• Campylobacter jejuni • Brucella abortus
obligate anaerobe	• Clostridium • Actinomyces
facultative anaerobe	most others

 Reactivation of tuberculosis usually appears in the better ventilated upper lobes of the lung!

2.6) <u>MOST COMMON CAUSES</u>

Many times, treatment cannot await the microbial lab results.
Choose your therapy based on your best guess of most common causes:

common cold	rhino viruses
pharyngitis, laryngitis	viral > bacterial (ß-hemolyzing Streptococci)
tonsillitis	ß-hemolyzing Streptococci
sinusitis	*Strep. pneumoniae, Staph. aureus*
otitis media	*Strep. pneumoniae, Hemophilus influenza*
bronchitis	*Hemophilus influenza, Strep. pneumoniae*
pneumonia - infants	**RSV**
- young adults	*Mycoplasma*
- elderly	*Strep. pneumoniae*
bacterial meningitis	
- neonates	*E. coli, Strep. agalactia, Listeria*
- children	*Neisseria meningitidis > Strep. pneumoniae*
- adults	**Strep. pneumoniae > Neisseria meningitidis**
aseptic meningitis	enteroviruses, arboviruses (Summer!)
endocarditis	*Strep. viridans*
post transfusion hepatitis	hepatitis C
carbuncle	*Staph. aureus*
sepsis (catheterized patient)	*Staph. aureus, Candida*
sepsis (burn wounds)	*Pseudomonas aeruginosa*
diarrhea - children	**Rotavirus**
- adults (US)	*Campylobacter*
- travelers	*E. coli, shigella, salmonella*
genital ulcer	herpes > syphilis
urethritis	*chlamydia > gonococcus*
cystitis	*E. coli*

Part B : Bacteria

2.7.) STAPHYLOCOCCI
(catalase +)

Staphylococci are Gram+ cocci that grow in grape-like clusters. Catalase is an enzyme that converts 2 H_2O_2 into 2 $H_2O + O_2$. Its presence distinguishes Staphylococci from Streptococci. Coagulase is specific for *Staph. aureus* and causes blood clotting.

	COAGULASE	NOVOBIOCIN	DISEASES
S. aureus	+		skin infections osteomyelitis endocarditis toxic shock syndrome food poisoning
S. epidermidis	-	sensitive	infections following: instrumentation implants etc.
S. saprophyticus	-	insensitive	urinary tract infections

Famous exotoxins:
- Enterotoxin A-F → diarrhea
- Toxic shock syndrome toxin → anaphylaxis
- Exfoliatin → scalded skin (hands and feet)
- Alpha toxin → tissue necrosis

Staph. aureus:
- *Colonizes anterior nares of most people.*
- *Community cases usually due to poor hygiene.*
- *Hospital cases usually involve patients who underwent invasive procedures.*
- *Survives drying - spread by hands of medical personnel.*

2.8.) <u>STREPTOCOCCI</u>

(catalase -)

Streptococci are Gram+ cocci that grow in chains. Compared to staphylococci, they grow better on enriched media and require a narrower temperature range. When grown on blood agar, they cause a characteristic pattern of RBC hemolysis which allows for a rough classification. Lancefield antigens determine the group and correlate better with pathogenicity.

	KEY FEATURES
ß-hemolytic streptococci complete hemolysis (clear halo)	*Strept. pyogenes* (Group A)[1] → pharyngitis → acute rheumatic fever → bacitracin sensitive other Strept. (Groups B-T)[1] → neonatal sepsis → meningitis → bacitracin insensitive

[1] *C-antigen, <u>c</u>ell-wall (=Lancefield antigen)*

"Strep throat":
- *acute sore throat*
- *malaise, fever (39° - 40°)*
- *yellow exudates on tonsils*
- *may need bacterial culture to distinguish from viral pharyngitis*

	KEY FEATURES
α-hemolytic streptococci incomplete hemolysis (green halo)	*Pneumococcus* → "classic" lobar pneumonia • capsule determines virulence (over 80 distinct serotypes) • bile soluble (lysis) • Optochin sensitive *Strept. viridans* → endocarditis • bile insoluble • Optochin insensitive
γ-hemolytic streptococci no hemolysis	**Enterococci (Group D)** → urinary tract infections

Enterococci are more resistant to antibiotics than other streptococci.

Famous exotoxins:
- Streptokinase
- Streptodornase (DNAse)
- Hyaluronidase
- Erythrogenic toxin
- Streptolysin O
- Streptolysin S

2.9.) NEISSERIA
bean-shaped, gram-negative diplococci

There are only 2 Neisseria species that cause human disease:

	KEY FEATURES
Meningococcus	<ul><li>has capsule</li><li>ferments maltose</li></ul><ul><li>meningitis (infants 6-24 months) [1]</li><li>Waterhouse-Friderichsen syndrome</li></ul><ul><li>Gram stain of CSF is diagnostic</li></ul><blockquote>➤ *TX:* penicillin G</blockquote>

Gonococcus	<ul><li>has pilus</li><li>does not ferment maltose</li></ul><ul><li>**male** : dysuria
	   purulent discharge</li><li>**female:** endocervical infections
	   salpingitis
	   infertility</li></ul><blockquote>➤ *TX:* - almost all resistant to penicillin
	  - ceftriaxone is drug of choice [2]</blockquote>

[1] "natural immunity" protects during the first 6 months of life, due to maternal IgG crossing the placenta.

[2] add tetracycline for coexisting *C. trachomatis* infection!

*Always suspect gonorrhea in adolescents and young adults
with purulent arthritis (common !)*

2.10.) <u>BACILLI</u>

<u>acid fast</u>
Mycobacteria

<u>non acid fast</u>

<u>GRAM-NEGATIVE</u>
E. coli
Salmonella
Shigella
Proteus
Pseudomonas
...

<u>GRAM-POSITIVE</u>

a) spore-forming

<u>aerobic</u>
Bacillus

<u>anaerobic</u>
Clostridium

b) non spore-forming

Listeria
Corynebacteria

"Bacilli" refers to any rod-shaped bacteria. The genus *Bacillus* specifically refers to Gram+ spore-forming aerobic rods.

2.11.) <u>GRAM-POSITIVE BACILLI</u>

	AEROBE	TOXINS	SPORES	
Bacillus anthracis	+	+	+	→ anthrax → woolsorter's disease → "fried rice" poisoning
Coryne-bacterium	+	+	-	→ diphtheria pseudomembranes Loeffler's telluride "Chinese characters"
Listeria	+	-	-	→ sepsis, meningitis neonates or immunosuppressed "Chinese characters" + motile!
Clostridium	-	+	+	→ tetanus → botulism → gas gangrene (α-toxin) → food poisoning (reheated meat) → pseudomembranous colitis
Lactobacillus	-	-	-	protects GI and vagina prefers acidic pH < 4.5

<u>PSEUDOMEMBRANOUS COLITIS</u>
(the usual suspects):
➤ clindamycin
➤ ampicillin
➤ cephalosporins

2.12.) <u>CLOSTRIDIA</u>

Clostridia are anaerobe spore-forming rods found in the soil, especially when fertilized with animal excreta.

	KEY FEATURES
Cl. botulinum	• motile • types A-G (antigenically different exotoxins)
Cl. tetani	• motile • 10 types (flagellar antigen) • but all have the same exotoxin

Cl. perfringens	• non-motile
	
	• **α-toxin** = lecithinase
	  → gas gangrene (soldiers)
	
	• **enterotoxin** (heat labile)
	  → food poisoning (reheated meat stews)

BOTULISM:
- *Cl. Botulinum* spores are highly resistant to heat, but toxins are not.
- Proper canning and heating of food prevents botulism.
- Nausea, vomiting and abdominal cramps usually precede the neurological symptoms: Dry mouth, diplopia, loss of pupillary reflexes, followed by descending paralysis and respiratory failure.

TETANUS:
- Toxin enters the CNS along the peripheral nerves
- Incubation period 5~10 days
- Stiffness of the jaws, difficulty swallowing, fever, headache
- *Risus sardonicus*: fixed "smile" and elevated eyebrows
- Severe spasms of neck, back and abdominal muscles
- Intact sensorium and CSF

2.13.) <u>ENTEROBACTERIACEAE</u>
(facultative anaerobe gram-negative rods)

Enterobacteriaceae are the most common cause of UTI and a major cause of diarrhea. They inhabit the lower GI tract of humans and animals and survive easily in free nature.

> 5 major genera. All look the same, some are motile, some are not. Differentiated by cultural appearance and biochemical activities. Subtyping is done by serology.

	LAB FEATURES	CLINICAL FEATURES
E. coli	motile lactose +	→ most common cause of UTI → neonatal meningitis [1]
Salmonella (1,500 species)	motile lactose - only *S. typhi* produces gas	food poisoning • poultry products • incubation 1~2 days enteric fever (typhoid, paratyphoid) • incubation 10~14 days
Shigella	non-motile lactose - no gas	dysenteriae (serious) flexneri, boydii, sonnei (mild) • watery diarrhea followed by fever, bloody stools and cramping

[1] maternal IgM are too big and do NOT cross placenta → no protection

Shigella is 1,000x more infective than Salmonella.

> <u>Treatment of salmonella infections:</u>
> **gastroenteritis:** fluid replacement, no antibiotics
> **typhoid:**   chloramphenicol, ampicillin

	LAB FEATURES	CLINICAL FEATURES
Proteus [1]	motile urease	**urinary tract infections** urease-production → ammonium calculi *Proteus* does NOT cause gastroenteritis
Klebsiella	non-motile encapsulated	**Community acquired:** - indistinguishable from "classic" lobar pneumonia - "currant jelly" sputum **Hospital acquired:** - UTI - respiratory tract infections - wound infections - **resistant to many antibiotics !!!**

[1] *has antigens that cross-react with anti-rickettsial antibodies (Weil-Felix reaction)*

> ***K-antigen:*** *capsule*
> ***H-antigen:*** *flagella*
> ***O-antigen:*** *surface*

Patients recovering from Salmonella gastroenteritis can shed the organism for many weeks or months. Be aware of chronic carriers who are food handlers!

2.14.) <u>MORE ENTEROBACTERIACEAE</u>

	KEY FEATURES
Bacteroides fragilis anaerobic	• most common cause of gram-negative abdominal infections • forms abscesses in organs or deep tissues ➤ *TX: metronidazole*
Vibrio cholera comma-shaped	• rice-watery diarrhea (non bloody) ➤ *TX: tetracycline*
Vibrio parahaemolyticus comma-shaped	• diarrhea from raw seafood (Sushi) ➤ *self-limited*
Campylobacter jejuni curved rods	• watery, foul smelling stools later may become bloody • most common cause of diarrhea in US ➤ *TX: erythromycin, aminoglycoside*
Helicobacter pylori very similar to Campylobacter (but urease +)	• gastritis • peptic ulcer • MALT lymphoma ➤ *TX: metronidazole + tetracycline + bismuth* *(three drug regimen)*

<u>*CHOLERA TOXIN:*</u>

ADP-ribosylates stimulatory G_s protein
(locks it in the "on"-state)
→ permanent activation of adenylate cyclase
→ secretory diarrhea

2.15.) <u>GRAM- BACILLI (ZOONOTIC)</u>

	KEY FEATURES

Yersinia pestis
bipolar staining
	bubonic plague
	    rodents → fleas → humans
	    large, very tender lymph nodes
	
	pulmonary plague
	    humans → humans
	
	➢ *TX: streptomycin, tetracycline*

Pasteurella	• wound infections (dog and cat bites) • cellulitis, osteomyelitis ➢ *TX: penicillin G*
Brucella	undulating fever • Br. abortus (cattle) • Br. melitensis (goats and sheep) • Br. suis (hogs) ➢ *TX: tetracycline, gentamycin*
Francisella	tularemia • rabbits → ticks → humans • influenza-like • large, tender lymph nodes ➢ *TX: streptomycin*

Plague ("Black Death") *killed 25 million people in Europe in the 14th Century. Today, 30-40 cases/year are reported in the US. Bubonic plague has up to 75% mortality, pneumonic plague has 100% mortality if untreated. Avoid sick or dead wild rodents!*

2.16.) OTHER GRAM- BACILLI

	KEY FEATURES
Pseudomonas	• easily survives in un-sterile water • musty odor, greenish bluish pus • common wound infection (especially burns) • pneumonia, UTI ➢ *resists most antibiotics and disinfectants !!!*
Hemophilus	• very small bacterium • requires blood (chocolate agar) for culture • dramatic decrease since vaccination • *H. influenza* : bronchitis, meningitis • *H. ducreyi* : chancroid
Bordetella	• pertussis toxin → whooping cough ➢ *TX: erythromycin (best during catarrhal stage!)*
Legionella *(aerobe)*	• gram-negative cell wall, but stains only faintly • found in any stagnant water • atypical pneumonia [1] • no cold agglutinins (unlike mycoplasma) ➢ *TX: erythromycin*

[1] clinical spectrum ranges from mild, self-limited to fatal Legionnaire's disease.

PERTUSSIS TOXIN:

ADP-ribosylates inhibitory G_i protein
(locks it in the "off"-state)
→ permanent activation of adenylate cyclase

2.17.) MYCOBACTERIA

About half of the World population is infected with M. tuberculosis. 30 million have active disease. Related to poverty, overcrowding and poor hygiene.

	KEY FEATURES
M. tuberculosis	• slow respiratory infection • primary lesion: Ghon complex • most morbidity is due to reactivation
M. bovis	• unpasteurized milk • GI tuberculosis

M. leprae	• grows at lower temp. than M. tuberculosis
	• found in nasal secretions and skin lesions
	• **tuberculoid leprosy:** granulomas
	                     skin test positive
	• **lepromatous leprosy:** nodular skin lesions
	                     skin test negative [1]

Atypical M. avium-intracellulare	 • clinically indistinguishable from tuberculosis • immunosuppressed patients (AIDS) ➤ *highly resistant to therapy !!!*
M. marinum	• causes tuberculosis in fish • "swimming pool granuloma" in humans

[1] *due to deficiency in cell-mediated immunity!*

TUBERCULOSIS:

Ghon complex: primary lesion in lung + calcified hilar lymph node

reactivation: favors upper lobes of lung
liquefying necrosis → cavity formation

miliary TBC: due to hematogenous spread of tubercle bacilli
(lesions resemble millet seeds)

2.18.) <u>HIGHER BACTERIA</u>

- gram-positive rods
- filamentous, branching growth: were confused with fungi in the past
- cause indolent, slowly progressive diseases

	KEY FEATURES
Actinomyces anaerobe	• growths in normal mouth flora <u>Lump jaw</u> • following tooth extraction • inflammatory sinuses → discharge to surface • sulfur granules ➢ *TX: penicillin* *surgical drainage*
Nocardia aerobe	• growths in soil <u>Subcutaneous tissue infections</u> • following minor trauma (outdoors) <u>Pulmonary infections</u> • inhalation of dust or soil ➢ *TX: sulfonamides* *surgical drainage*

2.19.) <u>SPIROCHETES</u>

	KEY FEATURES
T. pallidum	• syphilis • related diseases: Yaws, Bejel, Pinta ➤ *TX: penicillin G*
B. burgdorferi	• Lyme disease • tick bite (mainly east coast) *TX: doxycycline, ceftriaxone, amoxicillin*
B. recurrentis	• relapsing fever • antigens undergo variations → relapses • human → louse or tick → human ➤ *TX: tetracycline*
L. interrogans	• leptospirosis • sewers, water contaminated with <u>rat urine</u> • fever, jaundice, hemorrhage, uremia ➤ *TX: penicillin G*

<u>LYME DISEASE</u>:
1.) primary lesion (3-30 days): - at site of tick bite
- expanding macule or papule with central clearing *(erythema migrans)*

2.) second stage (weeks - months): - cardiac AV block
- fluctuating meningitis
- facial palsy
- peripheral neuropathy

3.) third stage (weeks - years): - arthritis of large joints (knee)

2.20.) CHLAMYDIA

Intracellular bacterium that cannot make ATP and cannot live outside.
Cell wall does not contain peptidoglycans.

	KEY FEATURES
C. pneumoniae	• "walking pneumonia" in young adults ➤ *TX: tetracycline*
C. trachomatis	<u>different strains cause different diseases</u> : • **urethritis** most common non-gonorrheal urethritis • **lymphogranuloma venereum** large and tender inguinal lymph nodes may drain pus through skin • **trachoma** chronic conjunctivitis that leads to blindness ➤ *TX: tetracycline*
C. psittaci	• **pneumonia** (sometimes plus hepatitis) from bird feces ➤ *TX: tetracycline*

 Giemsa stain shows typical cytoplasmic inclusions in epithelial cells.

LIFE CYCLE OF CHLAMYDIAE:
→ elementary body infects cell (attaches to cell membrane)
→ enters cell by endocytosis
→ elementary body then transforms into large reticulate body (visible cytoplasmic inclusions)
→ reticulate body condenses and forms many new elementary bodies that are released when cell ruptures

2.21.) RICKETTSIA

		VECTOR	RESERVOIR
Typhus: epidemic [1] endemic [2] scrub [3]	R. prowazekii R. typhi R. tsutsugamushi	lice fleas mite	humans rodents rodents
Rocky Mountain spotted fever	R. rickettsiae	ticks	dogs, rodents
Q fever	C. burnetii	transmitted by inhalation (slaughterhouses)	cattle, sheep
Trench fever	R. quintana	lice	humans

[1] war, famine, crowding, infrequent bathing (no cases in US since WW II)
[2] murine typhus, 30-60 cases/year in US (mostly Texas)
[3] Southeast Asia, Japan

 Treatment for all rickettsial infections: tetracycline

Part C : Viruses

2.22.) <u>DNA VIRUSES</u>

➤ All DNA viruses have a double stranded genome, except parvoviruses.
➤ All DNA viruses have an icosahedral nucleocapsid, except poxviruses.
➤ Pox are the largest and most complex viruses.

FAMILY	VIRUS	DISEASES
Parvo	B19	• erythema infectiosum, (5th disease) "slapped cheek" appearance
Papova	Papilloma	• genital warts → cervix carcinoma multiply in squamous cells
	JC	• leukoencephalopathy (in immunocompromised patients)
Adeno	~100 serotypes	• respiratory infections • atypical pneumonia o conjunctivitis o gastroenteritis o hemorrhagic cystitis
Pox	Variola	• smallpox has been eradicated
	Vaccinia	• cowpox
	Molluscum contagiosum	• small pink warts of skin
Hepadna	HBV	• serum hepatitis B liver cell carcinoma

Vaccinia is serologically related to Variola, but the origin of this virus (recombinant of smallpox and cowpox?) is unknown.

2.23.) <u>HERPES VIRUSES</u>
(double stranded DNA)

All Herpes viruses produce an initial overt infection followed by a period of latency.
Reactivation of virus in immunocompromised host results in recurrent infection.

VIRUS	DISEASES	during latency the virus rests in:
HSV1 HSV2	• mainly oral herpes • mainly genital herpes - both multiply in fibroblasts	trigeminal ganglion sacral DRG
VZV	• chickenpox, shingles	thoracolumbar DRG [1]
EBV	• infectious mononucleosis o Burkitt's lymphoma (Africa) o nasopharyngeal carcinoma (China)	B lymphocytes
CMV	• cytomegalic inclusion disease heterophil negative mononucleosis (no pharyngitis !)	leukocytes
HHV-6	• roseola (6th disease)	T lymphocytes
HHV-8	• Kaposi sarcoma	unknown

[1] DRG = dorsal root ganglion: eruptions follow sensory nerve distribution!

Chickenpox: lesions appear in <u>different</u> stages of evolution
(vesicular → pustular → crusts)

Smallpox: lesions appear in <u>same</u> stage of evolution

2.24.) <u>RNA VIRUSES</u>

80% of respiratory tract infections are viral. The most important are influenza (RNA), parainfluenza (RNA), rhinovirus (RNA) and adenovirus (DNA).

FAMILY	VIRUS	DISEASES
Picorna	**Rhino**	• **common cold**
	Echo	• meningitis, URI, diarrhea
	Hepatitis A	• infectious hepatitis A
	Polio	• paralysis (α-motoneuron)
	Coxsackie A	• herpangina
		• hand/foot/mouth disease
	Coxsackie B	• myocarditis
		• Bornholm disease
Reo	Rota	• gastroenteritis (children)
Orthomyxo	Influenza A, B, C	• **influenza**
		H antigen: hemagglutinin
		N antigen: neuraminidase
Paramyxo	Rubeola	• measles
		• encephalitis
		• SSPE
	Parainfluenza	• **croup** (subglottitis)
	Mumps	• parotitis, orchitis
	RSV	• bronchiolitis, pneumonia
Toga	Rubella	• German measles
	Arbo	• encephalitis

Antigenic drift: ***"drift along"*** (mutation within H_2N_2)
  - subtle changes of H or N antigens
  - caused by point mutations of viral RNA

Antigenic shift: ***"shift gears"*** ($H_2N_2 \rightarrow H_3N_2$)
  - severe epidemics / pandemics
  - caused by gene recombination

2.25.) <u>ARBO VIRUSES</u>
(arthropod borne)

Arboviruses cause seasonal disease transmitted by insects (arthropods). Reservoir are birds and small mammals.

FAMILY	VIRUS	DISEASES	VECTOR
Toga	Alphavirus	• EEE • WEE	mosquito
Flavi	Flavivirus	• St. Louis encephalitis • yellow fever • Dengue fever	mosquito
Bunya	Bunyavirus	• California encephalitis	mosquito
	Hantavirus	• fulminant respiratory infection	deer mice
Reo	Orbivirus	• Colorado tick fever	tick

 ***Hantavirus** is an exception among Arboviruses: no arthropod vector!*

2.26.) <u>SLOW VIRAL DISEASES OF CNS</u>

Slowly progressing neurologic diseases due to viral persistence.

> ➤ personality changes
> ➤ intellectual deterioration
> ➤ autonomic or motor dysfunctions

AIDS dementia complex	HIV
subacute sclerosing panencephalitis	measles virus
progressive multifocal leukoencephalopathy	JC virus

2.27.) <u>PRIONS</u>

<u>Prions are infectious proteins:</u>
o   can be transmitted to other species (chimpanzees, mice etc.)
   by inoculation of infected brain tissue
o   are NOT transmitted by body secretions
   (no risk for medical personnel and care givers)
o   are NOT inactivated by formalin!

Kuru ("trembling disease")	humans
Creutzfeldt-Jakob	humans
Scrapie	sheep
BSE ("mad cow disease")	cattle

 Scrapie is not transmitted to humans. BSE may occasionally cause a variant of Creutzfeldt-Jacob disease.

2.28.) <u>RETROVIRUSES</u>

Single stranded RNA viruses encode a reverse transcriptase (RNA-dependent DNA polymerase that copies the virus genome into the host genome):

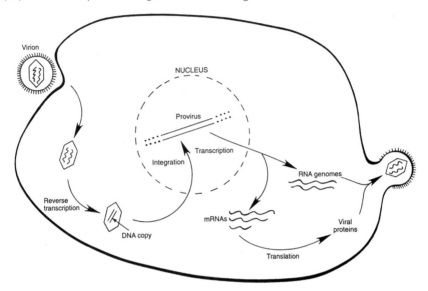

From *Sherris Medical Microbiology*, 3rd edition, p. 544, edited by Kenneth J. Ryan.
Copyright 1994 by Appleton&Lange, Norwalk, Connecticut. Used with permission.

Two main groups: (onco=tumor, lenti=slow)

oncoviruses	HTLV-1	adult T-cell leukemia
lentiviruses	HIV-1 HIV-2	AIDS

HTLV-1 simply activates existing cellular genes (c-onc = protooncogenes) resulting in malignant transformation.
Other retroviruses cause tumors (in animals) by expressing viral oncogenes (v-onc) or inserting promoters or enhancers in the vicinity of proto-oncogenes (c-onc).

2.29.) <u>HIV</u>

HIV is the causative agent of AIDS. HIV-1 is the most common and many subtypes have been found depending on geographic location. HIV-2 (West-Africa) is much less common and less virulent. It may give "false negative" on the usual ELISA test. The genome of HIV contains only 3 major genes: env, gag, and pol:

genome	• two identical single strands of RNA (both have positive polarity, cannot form double strand!)
env	• **gp41** : mediates cell fusion • **gp120** : binds to CD4 receptor (mutates rapidly !) gp = glycoproteins in lipid envelope
gag	• core capsid protein: **p24 (serologic marker)**
pol	• reverse transcriptase • integrase • protease
tat	• regulatory portion of genome • increases rate of transcription • also suppresses synthesis of class I MHC proteins

<u>Tests for HIV antibodies:</u>

ELISA: - good sensitivity, good specificity
- for screening

Western blot: - extremely specific
- to confirm a positive ELISA

 Antibodies are not detectable for 2-4 weeks after infection.

Part D : Fungi & Parasites

2.30.) FUNGI

WHAT THEY LOOK LIKE:

- Fungi come it two forms: **yeasts (=single cells)** and **molds (=forming hyphae)**
- Most fungi can be both (i.e. are dimorphic). Typically they form yeasts at 37°C and molds if they grow outside the human body.

EXAMPLES:

MOLDS	DIMORPHIC FUNGI	YEASTS
aspergillus • farmer's lung	histoplasma • pulmonary infection	candida • thrush, vaginitis
	blastomyces • respiratory tract infection	cryptococcus • pneumonia, meningitis
	coccidioides • desert rheumatism	

MOLDS:

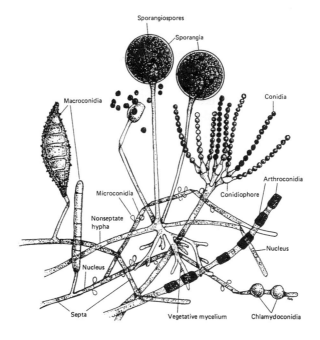

YEASTS:

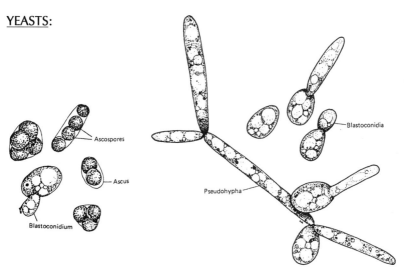

From *Sherris Medical Microbiology*, 3rd edition, p. 574, edited by Kenneth J. Ryan.
Copyright 1994 by Appleton&Lange, Norwalk, Connecticut. Used with permission.

115

HOW THEY REPRODUCE:

- Fungi reproduce in two manners : Sexual and asexual.
- Most fungi can do both (i.e. fungi perfecti).
- Fungi that do not reproduce sexually are called fungi imperfecti.
  (or maybe they "couple" so rarely, that their spores went undetected so far)

- **Sexual reproduction:**   2 cells fuse, diploid cell divides by meiosis
- **Asexual reproduction:** haploid cell divides by mitosis (like bacteria)

---

spores (sexual): Ascospores, Basidiospores, Zygospores etc.
conidia (asexual): Arthroconidia, Chlamydioconidia etc.

Note how both yeasts and molds can produce spores and conidia:

	YEASTS	MOLDS
asexual	Blastoconidia (= "buds") Pseudohyphae	Arthroconidia Chlamydioconidia
sexual	Ascospores	Basidiospores Zygospores

2.31.) <u>FUNGAL DISEASES</u>

Clinically, fungi most often cause skin disease, but some can cause systemic infections. Immunocompromised patients may develop opportunistic fungal disease. Diagnosis is made by light microscopy using 10% KOH, which dissolves tissue but not fungal walls:

		MICROSCOPIC FEATURES
cutaneous	• dermatophytosis (ringworm)	o hyphae
	• tinea versicolor	o hyphae
subcutaneous	• mycetoma	o "tree" shaped (sporangia)
	• sporotrichosis	o cigar shaped budding yeast
systemic	• coccidioidomycosis	o soil: arthrospores tissue: endospores
	• histoplasmosis	o yeasts in macrophages
	• blastomycosis	o broad based bud with double refractory walls
opportunistic	• cryptococcosis	o capsule on India ink prep.
	• candidiasis	o pseudohyphae germ tubes
	• aspergillosis	o V shaped

Histoplasmosis: - humid soil (Mississippi river)
- most infections are asymptomatic
- progressive pulmonary disease resembles tuberculosis

Coccidioidomycosis: - "valley fever": fever, cough, arthralgia
- endemic to Arizona, Nevada, New Mexico.

Aspergillosis: - allergy, exacerbates asthma
- pulmonary disease (immunocompromised patients)
- radiologically visible fungus ball within cavity

2.32.) <u>MALARIA</u>

Malaria is found in most tropical areas and more than 1 million children die of the disease each year. Sporozoa are unique intracellular protozoa that cycle through sexual and asexual places of reproduction:

> **Mosquito: sexual cycle →** forms sporozoites
> **Human:** asexual cycle → forms schizonts

1.) **Sporozoites** are introduced into blood
2.) Exo-erythrocytic phase: sporozoites differentiate into merozoites
3.) **Merozoites** settle in liver (latent forms called hypnozoites)
4.) Liver releases merozoites
5.) Merozoites infect red blood cells
6.) Ring-shaped **trophozoite** matures, forms multinucleated schizonts
7.) RBC releases either 10-20 new merozoites or **gametocytes**

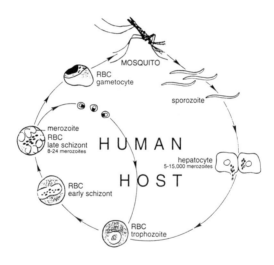

From *Sherris Medical Microbiology*, 3rd edition, p. 644, edited by Kenneth J. Ryan.
Copyright 1994 by Appleton&Lange, Norwalk, Connecticut. Used with permission.

Sporozoites reproduce asexually inside RBCs. Eventually the RBCs burst, causing periodic fever and anemia in the patient.

	KEY FEATURES
Vivax	• fever peak every 48 h • latent liver forms • very common
Ovale	• fever peak every 48 h • latent liver forms • rare
Falciparum	• fever peak every 48 h • most severe, life threatening • no trophozoites/schizonts found in blood • banana shaped gametocytes
Malariae	• fever peak every 72 h

Prevention:
1. mosquito screens, repellents
2. mefloquine or doxycycline when traveling to areas where chloroquine-resistance is common.

2.33.) TISSUE PROTOZOA

A) LATENT INFECTION IN MOST PEOPLE:

Pneumocystis carinii	• probably a fungus, (antifungal drugs are ineffective!) • common in **AIDS** patients • sudden onset fever, dyspnea, tachypnea ➤ *TX: trimethoprim-sulfamethoxazole* *pentamidine*
Toxoplasma gondii	• natural host: GI tract of cats • cat feces, undercooked meat (pork) • cysts → invade gut wall → muscles, brain • severe **congenital defects** if pregnant woman gets infected ➤ *TX: sulfonamide (first trimester)* *sulfonamide-pyrimethamine (all others)*

B) TROPICAL/SUBTROPICAL: (transmitted by insects)

Leishmania	
a) L. donovani	a) Kala-Azar (visceral) "black sickness" (GI bleeding)
b) L. brasiliensis	b) Espundia (mucocutaneous ulcers)
c) L. mexicana, L. tropica	c) cutaneous leishmaniosis (red papule, satellites, ulcerating) ➤ *TX: sodium stibogluconate*
Trypanosoma	
a) T. cruzi (America)	a) kissing bug: **Chagas disease** ➤ *TX: nifurtimox*
b) T. gambiense (Africa)	b) Tsetse fly: **sleeping sickness**
c) T. rhodesiense (Africa)	c) more severe than T. gambiense ➤ *TX: suramin, melarsoprol*

2.34.) INTESTINAL PROTOZOA

Protozoa cause bloody diarrhea if they invade the wall of the GI tract. If they don't invade, the stool will be non-bloody. Interference with fat absorption results in greasy, foul-smelling stools that may float on water.

Entamoeba histolytica	• cysts have 4 nuclei • bloody, mucus, diarrhea • liver abscess • can be sexually transmitted ➤ *TX: metronidazole*
Giardia lamblia (most common)	• cyst: 4 nuclei • trophozoite: 2 nuclei, 4 pairs of flagella (looks like a clown....) • excystation in duodenum • non-bloody, foul smelling diarrhea ➤ *TX: metronidazole*
Cryptosporidium	• excystation in small intestine • trophozoites do not invade gut wall • severe diarrhea in immunocompromised (AIDS!) ➤ *no effective therapy*

2.35.) TRICHOMONAS
very common sexually transmitted disease

Trichomonas	• 1 nucleus, 4 flagella, undulating membrane • male : asymptomatic or non-purulent urethritis • female: foul-smelling, watery, green discharge ➤ *TX: metronidazole*

2.36.) <u>FLUKES</u>
(Trematodes)

A) <u>BLOOD FLUKES</u>: (Schistosoma)

Intermediate host is a snail that releases larvae (cercariae) which can penetrate human skin. They enter small veins, pass through the right heart and lungs into the systemic circulation. After passing through intestinal capillaries, they settle in the portal vein where they mature to sexually active adults.

	ROUTE OF INFECTION:	EVENTUALLY SETTLES IN:
Sch. mansoni	penetrates skin	veins of colon
Sch. japonicum	penetrates skin	veins of small intestine
Sch. hematobium	penetrates skin	veins of urinary bladder

B) <u>TISSUE FLUKES</u>: (endemic to South East Asia)

	ROUTE OF INFECTION:	EVENTUALLY SETTLES IN:
Clonorchis sinensis	eating raw fish	**liver** → bile stones → bile obstruction → bile duct carcinoma
Paragonimus	eating raw crab meat	**lung** → eosinophilic inflammation

 Praziquantel eliminates flukes.

2.37.) <u>TAPEWORMS</u>
(Cestodes)

Long, ribbonlike worms that are the largest and most repulsive of intestinal parasites. If the patient ingested larvae, he becomes the primary host and the worms remain in the lumen of the gut. If the patient ingested eggs, he becomes as intermediate host: developing larvae invade the tissues and cause serious disease.

	SOURCE	INGESTED FORM	EVENTUALLY SETTLES IN:
T. solium [1]	pork	larvae	intestine
T. solium	human feces	eggs	brain, eyes (cysticerci)
T. saginata [2]	beef	larvae	intestine
D. latum	raw fish	larvae	intestine
Echinococcus	dog feces	eggs	in liver, lung, brain (cysts)

[1] *max. length: 5m*   [2] *max. length: 10m*

 Niclosamide eliminates tapeworms.

2.38.) <u>ROUNDWORMS</u>
(Nematodes)

Intestinal nematodes are found in soil where human feces are deposited or used as fertilizer. Severity of disease depends on worm load and tissue invasion.

A) <u>INGESTED FORM: EGGS</u>

Enterobius	perianal pruritus (at night)
Ascaris	worm lives in colon, larvas migrate to lung

B) <u>INGESTED FORM: LARVAE</u>

Necator	intestinal blood loss
Strongyloides	larvas penetrate skin, then migrate to lung
Trichinella	pork meat, larvae form cysts in striated muscle

C) <u>TRANSMITTED BY INSECT BITE</u>:

Wuchereria	microfilariae found in blood adult worm lives in lymph nodes → lymph obstruction
Onchocerca	"river blindness" microfilariae in subcutaneous tissue and eye

 Mebendazole and pyrantel pamoate eliminate roundworms.

PHARMACOLOGY

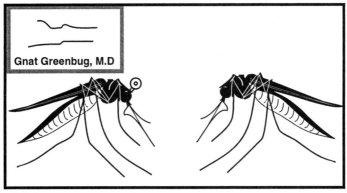

"Chemotherapy will increase your lifespan about
10 minutes, Mr. Mosley, which is not bad, given
your normal life cycle of 2 days."

3.1.) <u>DRUG INTERACTIONS</u>

Drug to drug interactions account for a significant number of adverse reactions. They can diminish or potentiate the desired effects, which is most serious for drugs with a low therapeutic index (sulfonylureas, tolbutamide). Interactions may involve absorption, distribution, metabolism and excretion of drugs or may be a more direct competition near the receptor site.

drugs that are easily displaced from albumins	• sulfonamides • phenylbutazone • tolbutamide • coumarin
drugs that induce P450	• alcohol • barbiturates • phenytoin • rifampicin
drugs that inhibit P450	• chloramphenicol • sulfonamides • phenylbutazone
drugs that compete for renal transporters	○ uric acid • probenecid • penicillins • sulfonamides • salicylates • thiazides

EXAMPLES:

(1) Risk of severe hemorrhage if coumarins are combined with any other drug that competes for albumin.

(2) Sulfonamides displace sulfonylureas from albumin → hypoglycemia

(3) Barbiturate induces P450 enzyme → enhanced metabolism of MAO inhibitors → ineffective treatment of depression.

(4) P450 induction → Enhanced estrogen metabolism → reduced oral contraceptive efficacy → unplanned pregnancy

(5) Steroids compete with MAO inhibitor for P450 enzyme → reduced metabolism of MAO inhibitor → risk of over dose

(6) Aspirin reduces renal secretion of uric acid and is contraindicated in gout.

3.2.) BAD COMBINATIONS

NEVER EVER COMBINE:	WITH THESE DRUGS:
aminoglycosides	• neuromuscular blockers (enhanced block) • loop diuretics (compounds ototoxicity)
MAO inhibitors	• levodopa (hypertensive crisis) • amphetamine (hypertensive crisis) • tricyclic antidepressants [1]
tricyclic antidepressants	• MAO inhibitors [1]

[1] *antidepressants should never be combined!*

3.3.) __FAMOUS SIDE EFFECTS__

There are at least as many questions on the USMLE about side effects of drugs as there are about main effects and mechanisms of action. Please study these very carefully!

FAMOUS SIDE EFFECT:	CAUSED BY:
anaphylactic shock	• penicillin • foreign proteins
hepatotoxicity	• isoniazid • halothane
renal toxicity	• phenacetin • other NSAIDs • cyclosporin
ototoxicity	• aminoglycosides
drug-induced lupus	• procainamide • hydralazine
photosensitivity (skin)	• tetracyclines • sulfonamides • sulfonylureas
cutaneous flushing	• niacin
hemolysis in patients with G6PD-deficiency	• sulfonamides • primaquine
bone marrow suppression	• chloramphenicol • ganciclovir • zidovudine (AZT)

3.4.) <u>ANTIDOTES</u>

Antitoxins are antibodies against bacterial toxins.
Antidotes interfere with the action or metabolism of toxic substances.

INTOXICATION	ANTIDOTE
acetaminophen	N-acetylcysteine
opiates	naloxone
benzodiazepines	flumazenil
methanol, ethylene glycol	ethanol
CO	100% O_2
cyanide	amyl nitrate
organophosphates	atropine, pralidoxime
iron	deferoxamine
lead	EDTA
coumarins	Vit. K
heparin	protamine

Intoxication with acidic drugs (e.g. barbiturate, salicylate):
Alkalinize urine (IV sodium-bicarbonate) to enhance renal excretion.

3.5.) <u>ANTIBIOTICS</u>

> **Bactericidal** drugs "kill" bacteria.
> **Bacteriostatic** drugs inhibit bacterial growth and require the
> host's immune system to "finish the job".

BACTERICIDAL	BACTERIOSTATIC
• penicillins	• chloramphenicol
• cephalosporins	• erythromycin
• aminoglycosides	• tetracyclines
• vancomycin	• sulfonamides
• quinolones	• trimethoprim

*Misuse of antibiotics results in emergence of antibiotic-resistant
strains. This creates an ever-increasing need for new drugs...*

GRAM-POSITIVE	GRAM-NEGATIVE	BROAD-SPECTRUM
• penicillin G	• aminoglycosides	• ampicillin
• vancomycin	• polymyxins	• cephalosporins
• bacitracin		• tetracyclines
		• chloramphenicol
		• sulfonamides

<u>MECHANISMS OF RESISTANCE</u>:

Bacteria become resistant to antibiotics if they acquire DNA coding for extra enzymes
(e.g. β-lactamase). There are 3 ways in which DNA may be acquired:

transduction	transmission of DNA by bacteriophages that carry plasmids (extrachromosomal DNA)
transformation	uptake and incorporation of DNA from environment
conjugation	direct transmission of DNA from cell to cell via sex pilus

3.6.) DRUGS OF CHOICE

Actinomyces	actinomycosis	penicillin G
Bacillus anthracis	anthrax	penicillin G
Bordetella pertussis	whooping cough	erythromycin
Borrelia Burgdorferi	Lyme disease	tetracycline
Campylobacter	acute inflammatory diarrhea	ciprofloxacin
Candida	vaginal candidiasis	miconazole
	systemic candidiasis	fluconazole
Chlamydia trachomatis	pelvic inflammatory disease	doxycycline
Chlamydia pneumoniae	pneumonia	tetracycline
H. influenza	pneumonia, meningitis	3rd gen. cephalosporin
Helicobacter pylori	gastric ulcer	metronidazole + tetracycline
Klebsiella	pneumonia	3rd gen. cephalosporin
	UTI	quinolones
Legionella	Legionnaire's disease	erythromycin
M. tuberculosis	tuberculosis	isoniazid + rifampin
		+ pyrazinamide + ethambutol
M. leprae	leprosy	dapsone + rifampin
M. pneumoniae	atypical pneumonia	erythromycin
N. gonorrhea	gonorrhea	ceftriaxone
N. meningitis	meningitis	penicillin G
Nocardia	pneumonia	trimethoprim/sulfamethoxazole
Proteus	UTI	quinolones
Rickettsia	spotted fever, end. typhus	tetracycline
Salmonella typhi	typhoid fever	trimethoprim/sulfamethoxazole
Shigella	dysentery	trimethoprim/sulfamethoxazole
Staph. aureus	skin infection	dicloxacillin
	sepsis, osteomyelitis	nafcillin or oxacillin
Strept. pyogenes	pharyngitis, erysipelas	penicillin G or V
Strept. viridans	endocarditis	penicillin + aminoglycoside
Treponema pallidum	syphilis	penicillin G
Trichomonas	trichomoniasis	metronidazole
Tropheryma whippelii	Whipple's disease	trimethoprim/sulfamethoxazole
Vibrio cholerae	cholera	tetracycline (+ fluids!)
Yersinia pestis	plague ("black death")	streptomycin

3.7.) PENICILLINS

Penicillin G is the drug of choice for *Streptococci* and non-penicillinase producing *Staphylococci*. Broad spectrum penicillins are similar to Pen. G but are also effective against some gram- bacteria. Extended spectrum penicillins are for *Pseudomonas*, but lose their effectiveness against gram+ infections.

narrow spectrum **β-lactamase sensitive**	penicillin G penicillin V	gram positive *Strept.*
β-lactamase resistant	methicillin oxacillin nafcillin cloxacillin	gram positive *Strept.*
broad spectrum	ampicillin amoxicillin	*Hemophilus* *Neisseria* *E. coli* *Proteus*
extended spectrum	carbenicillin	*Pseudomonas*

SIDE-EFFECTS:
- allergic reactions (maculopapular rash)
- cross-reactivity with cephalosporins!
- diarrhea (disruption of normal flora)

β-LACTAMASE (arrow indicates site of action):

penicillin   **cephalosporin**

3.8.) <u>CEPHALOSPORINS</u>

Cephalosporins were developed as penicillin alternative. They are relatively safe and the newer generations have a broader spectrum against gram- bacteria.

1st Generation (against gram-positive plus E. coli, Klebsiella)

cefazolin	longest half life
cephalexin	acid stable (oral administration)

2nd Generation (broader spectrum against gram-negative bacilli)

cefamandole	☹ disulfiram like reaction with ethanol bleeding (anti vitamin K action)
cefoxitin	potent against anaerobes (bowel perforation → E. coli, Bacteroides fragilis)

3rd Generation (superior activity against enterobacteriaceae)

cefotaxime	CNS permeable (Hemophilus meningitis!)
ceftriaxone	drug of choice for penicillin resistant gonorrhea

> **SIDE-EFFECTS:**
> Avoid in patients with known penicillin allergy.
> (significant cross reactivity)

3.9.) <u>ANTIVIRAL DRUGS</u>

Many of the antiviral drugs resemble nucleosides and take advantage of differences between eukaryotic DNA-polymerase and viral polymerases. Other drugs inhibit viral enzymes needed for assembly.

	MECHANISM OF ACTION	USED TO TREAT
amantadine	impairs uncoating	influenza A
interferons	inhibits viral multiplication	leukemia Kaposi sarcoma genital warts hepatitis B and C
ribavirin	guanosine analog	RSV infections in children
acyclovir	guanine analog, depends on viral thymidine kinase	HSV-1, HSV-2, VZV
vidarabine	adenosine analog	all Herpes group viruses
idoxuridine	thymidine analog	Herpes simplex keratitis
ganciclovir	like acyclovir	CMV
AZT	thymidine analog	HIV
protease inhibitors	inhibit cleavage of the gag-pol polyprotein → noninfectious virus particles	HIV

AZT: 3'-azido-3'-deoxythymidine

3.10.) ANTIFUNGAL DRUGS

Most antifungal drugs interact with sterols in the fungus cell membrane, forming large pores. They are quite toxic and side-effects are common.

imidazoles	• broad spectrum anti-fungals • itraconazole and fluconazole have replaced the more toxic ketoconazole
amphotericin B, itraconazole	• for severe systemic fungal infections
nystatin powder	• candida skin infections
griseofulvin	• given orally but accumulates in keratin • dermatophytic Infections

SIDE-EFFECTS:
Griseofulvin: hepatotoxic, teratogenic
Amphotericin: nephrotoxic, anemia
Nystatin, miconazole: systemic toxicity
(used only topically)

3.11.) ANTI-PROTOZOAL DRUGS

A) MALARIA:

Treatment of malaria requires destruction of (1.) erythrocyte schizont, (2.) erythrocyte gamete and (3.) liver schizont to prevent relapse.

prophylaxis	mefloquine or doxycycline
therapy	chloroquine
therapy *P. falciparum* [1]	quinine + pyrimethamine/sulfadoxine
prevention of relapse	primaquine [2]

[1] *usually resistant to chloroquine*
[2] *eradicates liver schizont of P. vivax and P. ovale*

B) OTHER PROTOZOA:

amebiasis (*Trichomonas, Chlamydia*)	metronidazole
leishmaniasis	stibogluconate
African sleeping sickness (*Trypanosoma gambiense*) (*Trypanosoma rhodesiense*)	melarsoprol / suramin
Chagas disease (*Trypanosoma cruzi*)	nifurtimox

3.12.) AIDS

A) TREATMENT OF HIV:

Combination of 2 to 4 drugs has become standard. This decreases the
likelihood of emergence of drug-resistant viral mutants.

		SIDE-EFFECTS
nucleosides	inhibit reverse transcriptase: • zidovudine (AZT) • didanosine (ddI)	• anemia, leukopenia • pancreatitis
non-nucleosides	inhibit reverse transcriptase: • Nevirapine (NVP)	• rashes
protease inhibitors	• Saquinavir (SAQ) • Indinavir (IND)	• kidney stones

B) TREATMENT OF OPPORTUNISTIC INFECTIONS:

Herpes simplex or zoster	acyclovir
CMV	ganciclovir
M. avium complex	clarithromycin + ethambutol
Candida (esophageal)	fluconazole, amphotericin B
Cryptococcus neoformans	fluconazole, amphotericin B
Pneumocystis carinii [1]	trimethoprim-sulfamethoxazole (pentamidine if allergic)
Toxoplasma gondii	pyrimethamine-sulfadiazine

[1] *prophylaxis necessary if CD4 < 200/μL*

3.13.) <u>INHIBITORS OF TRANSLATION</u>

RNA → Protein

A) <u>PROKARYOTES:</u>

Antibiotics selectively act on prokaryotic ribosomes (30S or 50S subunit):

	ACTS ON:	MECHANISM OF ACTION
aminoglycosides	30 S	inhibits initiation (binding of tRNA$_{fm}$)
tetracyclines	30 S	inhibits binding of all other tRNAs
chloramphenicol	50 S	inhibits peptidyl transferase
erythromycin	50 S	inhibits translocation

B) <u>EUKARYOTES:</u>

Chemicals that act on eukaryotic ribosomes (40S and 60S) are toxic and have no clinical use:

	ACTS ON:	MECHANISM OF ACTION:
lectins	40/60 S	inhibits initiation
cycloheximide	60 S	inhibits peptidyl transferase
diphtheria toxin	60 S	inhibits elongation factor
puromycin		incorporated into peptide chain → premature chain termination (eukaryotes and prokaryotes)

138

3.14.) INHIBITORS OF REPLICATION
DNA → DNA

Most of these drugs interfere with replication of eukaryotic cells
and are used for cancer treatment:

A) ANTI-FOLATES:

	MECHANISM OF ACTION	CLINICAL USE
methotrexate	mammalian folate synthesis	anticancer drug
trimethoprim	bacterial folate synthesis	antibiotic
pyrimethamine	protozoal folate synthesis	antimalarial

B) PURINE ANALOGS:

6-mercaptopurine	inhibits de novo synthesis	---
azathioprine	derivative of mercaptopurine	immunosuppressant

C) PYRIMIDINE ANALOGS:

cytarabine (ara-CTP)	incorporated into DNA	anticancer drug
5-fluorouracil	inhibits thymidylate synthesis	anticancer drug

D) ANTIBIOTIC CYTOTOXINS:

actinomycin D	binds to DNA	anticancer drug
doxorubicin	intercalates between base pairs	anticancer drug
bleomycin	causes strand breaks in DNA	anticancer drug

3.15.) <u>INHIBITORS OF TRANSCRIPTION</u>

DNA → RNA

A) <u>PROKARYOTES</u>:

rifampin	• binds to bacterial DNA-dependent RNA polymerase
	• inhibits initiation of RNA synthesis
	• anti-tuberculosis

B) <u>EUKARYOTES</u>:

α-amanitin	• blocks eukaryotic polymerase II
	• mushroom poison
actinomycin D	• binds to DNA
	• inhibits transcription (low concentration)
	• inhibits replication (high concentration)
	anticancer drug
doxorubicin	• intercalates between base pairs
	• inhibits translation and replication
	anticancer drug

3.16.) COMBINATION CHEMOTHERAPY

"Famous combinations":

ALL	prednisone vincristine
Wilms' tumor	dactinomycin vincristine
Hodgkin's disease	M mechlorethamine O vincristine P prednisone P procarbazine

☹ SPECIFIC SIDE EFFECTS:

doxorubicin	cardiotoxic
bleomycin	pulmonary fibrosis
cisplatin	renal toxicity
cyclophosphamide	hemorrhagic cystitis
vincristine	peripheral neuropathy
L-asparaginase	allergic reactions

Cycle-specific drugs:
antimetabolites, bleomycin, vinca alkaloids

3.17.) NSAIDs

NSAIDs decrease prostaglandin synthesis by inhibiting the key enzyme cyclooxygenase (COX). COX-1 controls many prostaglandins under "normal" conditions while COX-2 is active during inflammation. Selective COX-2 inhibitors have fewer side-effects than traditional NSAIDs.

GENERAL USE NSAIDs:

	MECHANISM OF ACTION	KEY FEATURES
aspirin	• acetylates cyclooxygenase	• **analgesic:** 600 mg/d • **anti-inflammatory**: 4g/d ☹ may cause Reye's syndrome ☹ contraindicated in gout !
acetaminophen	• no anti-inflammatory action • prefers CNS cyclooxygenase	• drug of choice for children with viral infections
ibuprofen	• similar spectrum as aspirin	• fewer GI side-effects
phenylbutazone	• anti-inflammatory • weak analgesic/antipyretic	• used when others have failed ☹ may cause skin rash, GI upset
indomethacin	• more potent anti-inflammatory than aspirin	• for acute gout • for ankylosing spondylitis ☹ may cause GI upset, pancreatitis
rofecoxib (Vioxx™)	• selective COX-2 inhibitor	• chronic pain (osteoarthritis)

Aspirin: Acetylation of platelet cyclooxygenase is irreversible!
→ don't give within 1 week prior to surgery!
→ don't give if patient has bleeding disorder
→ be careful with heparin!

SALICYLATE INTOXICATION:
mild: tinnitus, central hyperventilation
severe: respiratory plus metabolic acidosis

SLOW-ACTING DRUGS FOR RHEUMATOID ARTHRITIS:
Slow-acting drugs are not useful for acute attacks but improve the course of this chronic disease.

	MECHANISM OF ACTION	KEY FEATURES
gold	• suppresses macrophages	• add when regular NSAIDs fail to suppress inflammation ⊗ dermatitis, aplastic anemia
D-penicillamine	• reduces rheumatoid factor	• when gold has failed or is too toxic ⊗ bone marrow suppression
methotrexate[1]	• folic acid antagonist	• when all else has failed ⊗ bone marrow suppression ⊗ liver failure

[1] *much lower dose than what is used for cancer therapy.*

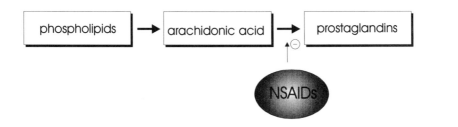

143

3.18.) <u>GOUT</u>

Acute or chronic arthritis that results from deposition of urate crystals in and around joints. Treatment of acute gout differs from that of chronic gout:

		MECHANISM OF ACTION
acute attack	colchicine	• inhibits migration of macrophages (depolymerizes microtubules) ☹ vomiting, abdominal pain
chronic gout	allopurinol	• purine analog • inhibits xanthine oxidase ☹ hypersensitivity reaction
chronic gout	probenecid	• blocks tubular secretion of penicillin [1] • blocks tubular reabsorption of uric acid

[1] *occasionally used to increase serum levels of antibiotics.*

> ### Causes of chronic gout:
> • elevated uric acid
> • Lesch-Nyhan syndrome
> • treatment of malignancies

 Most people with elevated uric acid levels do NOT have gout !

3.19.) ANTIHYPERTENSIVE DRUGS

Before treating a patient with "essential" hypertension, you need to rule out specific causes:
(1.) renal diseases, (2.) aldosteronism, (3.) coarctation of aorta, (4.) pheochromocytoma.
Choice of drug depends on clinical setting and contraindications:

	CLINICAL SETTING	CONTRAINDICATIONS
Ca^{2+} channel blockers	• for all patients	• congestive heart failure
β-blockers	• angina pectoris • post MI	• diabetes • asthma • peripheral vascular disease
thiazides	• congestive heart failure • chronic renal failure	• diabetes • hyperlipidemia
ACE inhibitors	• for all patients	• pregnancy

Hypertensive crisis: -sodium nitroprusside is rapid and potent.
- use only in hospital-setting.

☹
> **SIDE-EFFECTS:**
> **β-blockers:** - depression, fatigue, lethargy
>   - increased plasma triglycerides
> **thiazides:** - hypokalemia
>   - hypercalcemia

3.20.) ANTI-ANGIOTENSINS

Renin converts angiotensinogen to Ang-I. Angiotensin converting enzyme (ACE) converts Ang-I to the biologically active Ang-II which acts on angiotensin receptors on smooth muscle as a very potent vasoconstrictor.

	KEY FEATURES
captopril	• ACE inhibitor • decreases angiotensin II • increases bradykinin
enalapril	• ACE inhibitor • more potent • longer half time
saralasin	• blocks angiotensin receptors (weak agonist)

 ACE inhibitors work particularly well in young, white patients.

3.21.) ERGOT ALKALOIDS

Ergot is a product of a fungus growing on rye and other grains.

	MECHANISM OF ACTION	INDICATIONS
ergotamine, methysergide	vasoconstriction	• to abort migraine attack • post partum hemorrhage (contracts uterus)
bromocriptine	inhibits prolactin release	• hyperprolactinemia (pituitary adenomas) • infertility

☹ *diarrhea, nausea, severe vasospasms*

3.22.) DIURETICS

Diuretics increase the rate of urine formation. More important than just the volume of urine is the net loss of solute which mobilizes edema fluid. Diuretics are classified by the site of their action on renal tubules:

		INDICATIONS	⊗ SIDE EFFECTS
carb. anhydrase inhibitors	acetazolamide	• weak diuretic • rarely used	• metabolic acidosis [1]
loop diuretics	furosemide, ethacrynic acid	• acute pulmonary edema • hypercalcemia	• ototoxicity • hypokalemia • hyperuricemia
thiazides	chlorothiazide, hydrochlorothiazide, chlorthalidone	• hypertension • mild congestive heart failure • urinary calcium stones • diabetes insipidus	• hypokalemia • hypercalcemia • hyperglycemia • hyperuricemia
potassium sparing	spironolactone, (aldosterone antagonist) amiloride, triamterene	• usually combined with thiazides or loop diuretics • secondary hyperaldosteronism	• gynecomastia • menstrual irregularity
osmotic diuretics	mannitol	• acute renal failure • not useful in conditions a/w Na^+ retention	

[1] useful to prevent "mountain sickness" (respiratory alkalosis).

3.23.) <u>ANTIANGINAL DRUGS</u>

Angina pectoris occurs when cardiac work and O2 demand exceed the ability of coronary arteries to supply oxygenated blood. Antianginal drugs relax smooth muscles and are potent vasodilators.

	KEY FEATURES
nitroglycerin	• low dose : dilates veins, reduces preload • high dose: also dilates arterioles, reflex tachycardia (angina may get worse)
isosorbide dinitrate	• orally active • less potent than nitroglycerin
nifedipine	• relaxes arterioles • best for Prinzmetal's angina (coronary artery spasm)
verapamil	• slows heart rate • effect partially overcome by reflex tachycardia

Nitroglycerin generates metHb (Fe^{3+}) which can bind toxic cyanide - useful as an antidote!

CLASSIC ANGINA	MYOCARDIAL INFARCTION
• substernal pain	• substernal pain → spreads to arms or jaw
• lasts < 10 minutes • relieved by rest and nitrates	• lasts > 30 minutes • not relieved by rest or nitrates

3.24.) <u>PLATELET AGGREGATION INHIBITORS</u>

Whether platelets aggregate or not depends on the balance of inhibitors (PGI_2) and activators (thromboxane A_2) acting on surface receptors. Activated platelets release serotonin, ADP and additional thromboxane A_2.

	MECHANISM OF ACTION
aspirin	• inhibits cyclooxygenase (blocks thromboxane A_2 synthesis)
sulfinpyrazone	• inhibits degranulation (serotonin, ADP) • prolongs platelet survival
dipyridamole	• phosphodiesterase inhibitor • increases cAMP → inhibits degranulation

Prostacyclin → increases platelet cAMP → inhibits degranulation
Thromboxane A_2 → activates platelets (IP_3, DAG) → degranulation

Platelets release ADP and thromboxane A_2 → activate other platelets

Used for:
- prophylaxis of transient ischemic attacks
- decrease mortality in postmyocardial patients

3.25.) ANTICOAGULANTS

Patients with deep vein thrombosis are placed on heparin (injectable, fast acting) to prevent pulmonary embolism. Coumarins are taken orally and anticoagulant effect develops slowly.

	MECHANISM OF ACTION	ANTAGONIST
heparin	• enhances activity of antithrombin III	protamine sulfate
warfarin dicumarol	• antagonist of vit. K (II, VII, IX, X)	vitamin K

> **Monitor therapy with anticoagulants:**
> Warfarin: prothrombin time (PT): extrinsic pathway
> Heparin: partial thromboplastin time (aPPT): intrinsic pathway

3.26.) THROMBOLYTICS

Thrombolytic drugs are used to dissolve blood clots (acute MI)

	MECHANISM OF ACTION	ANTAGONIST
streptokinase	• derived from streptococci • activates plasminogen (plasmin then degrades fibrin)	aminocaproic acid
urokinase	• derived from human fetal renal cells • less antigenicity than streptokinase	
TPA	• "fibrin selective" [1]	

[1] activates only plasminogen already bound to fibrin

3.27.) <u>ANTIARRHYTHMIC DRUGS</u>

All antiarrhythmic drugs have the potential to induce arrhythmias. Therapy sometimes is a matter of "trial and error". These drugs are classified by their action on the cardiac action potential:

class 1	Na^+ channel blockers
class 2	β-blockers
class 3	K^+ channel blockers
class 4	Ca^{2+} channel blockers

CLASS	DRUGS	APD	UV	INDICATIONS
1A	quinidine, procainamide	↑	↓	• ectopic arrhythmias
1B	lidocaine, phenytoin	↓	↓	• acute ventricular flutter/fibrillation • digitalis induced arrhythmias
1C	flecainide encainide	∅	↓	• "broad spectrum" antiarrhythmic
2	propanolol			• atrial tachycardia • post MI (prophylactic)
3	bretylium amiodarone			• severe unresponsive ventricular arrhythmias
4	verapamil			• atrial tachycardia • atrial flutter

ADP: Action potential duration   *UV:* Upstroke velocity

☹
SIDE-EFFECTS:
procainamide: reversible lupus erythematosus
phenytoin: gingiva hyperplasia
quinidine: potentiates digitoxin toxicity

3.28.) INOTROPIC DRUGS

increased strength of cardiac contractions → increased stroke volume

Cardiac glycosides derived from the foxglove plant inhibit Na^+/K^+ ATPase. Increased intracellular Na^+ levels decrease Na^+/Ca^{2+} exchanger, resulting in elevated Ca^{2+} and stronger muscle contraction (positive inotropic effect).

		KEY FEATURES
glycosides	digoxin, digitoxin	• glycosides have a low therapeutic index!!! • digoxin: short, digitoxin: long action
β-agonists	dobutamine, dopamine	• β-agonists increase cAMP • less tachycardia or peripheral side effects than isoproterenol or epinephrine
PDE inhibitors	amrinone	☹ thrombocytopenia
	milrinone	☺ does not affect platelets

 Dopamine enhances renal blood flow and is particularly useful for treatment of shock.

GLYCOSIDE SIDE-EFFECTS:
extracardiac: - nausea, abdominal pain
- fatigue
- confusion, disorientation
- color misperception: yellow
cardiac: - AV block, arrhythmias

Toxicity of glycosides is enhanced by:
➢ hypokalemia
➢ alkalosis
➢ hypoxia
➢ hypothyroidism

3.29.) ASTHMA

Asthma is due to type I hypersensitivity reaction of the airways. Treatment aims at relaxing bronchial smooth muscles and reducing airway inflammation:

DRUG	INDICATION	MECHANISM OF ACTION
metaproterenol, terbutaline, albuterol	mild, intermittent asthma	β_2-selective agonists
theophylline	more severe asthma	phosphodiesterase inhibitor → cAMP ↑
cromolyn	prophylaxis	stabilizes mast cells
corticosteroids (inhaled)	severe, chronic asthma	anti-inflammatory
corticosteroids I.V.	status asthmaticus	anti-inflammatory

SIDE-EFFECTS:
β_2-**agonists:** - tremor
             - dizziness, palpitations
theophylline: - arrhythmias, seizures

Avoid common triggers: dust mites, molds, pollen…

3.30.) <u>INSULINS</u>

for treatment of IDDM = type 1

Hyperglycemia is responsible for most of the long-term complications of diabetes. Therapy attempts to lower HbA_{1C} (indicator of glucose during preceding 1-3 months) while avoiding hypoglycemic reactions.

		PEAK	DURATION
CZI	"regular insulin"	30 min	120 min
semilente	given subcutaneously rapid onset	2-3 h	5-8 h
lente	mix of semi and ultra	8-12 h	18-24 h
ultralente	prolonged action	14-20 h	36 h
PZI	CZI treated with protamine	24 h	36 h

Human insulin made by recombinant DNA techniques is preferred because it is less antigenic.

SIDE-EFFECTS:
hypoglycemia: sweating, anxiety, tremor, weakness
allergy: beef > pork > human insulin
fat atrophy: at site of injection

A common schedule:
- mix CZI and NPH (lente)
- give twice daily (morning and evening)
- monitor glucose in morning and afternoon

3.31.) <u>SULFONYLUREAS</u>

for treatment of NIDDM = type 2

Sulfonylureas lower plasma glucose by stimulating insulin secretion. They block K^+ channels of β-pancreatic cells, leading to membrane depolarization, increased intracellular Ca^{2+} and insulin secretion.

	DURATION OF ACTION
tolbutamide	8 h
glyburide, glipizide	20 h, most potent
chlorpropamide	48 h

Sulfonylureas are contraindicated in patients with liver or kidney failure: Accumulation will increase risk of hypoglycemia (especially with chlorpropamide)

Sulfonylureas are tightly bound to albumin. Competition with other albumin-binding drugs results in dangerous hypoglycemia.

3.32.) <u>HYPERLIPIDEMIAS</u>

Hyperlipidemia increases the risk of coronary artery disease – "good" cholesterol (HDL) lowers the risk, "bad" cholesterol (LDL) increase the risk. Here is how to calculate LDL from measurement of other blood lipids:

LDL = Total Cholesterol - HDL - (Triglycerides / 5)

TYPES OF HYPERLIPIDEMIA:

	ELEVATED FRACTION	DEFECT
Type I	chylomicrons *(triglycerides)*	lipoprotein lipase
Type IIA	LDL *(cholesterol)*	LDL receptor
Type IIB	LDL *(cholesterol)* VLDL *(triglycerides)*	mutant apoprotein ?
Type III	IDL *(triglycerides and cholesterol)*	mutant apoprotein E
Type IV	VLDL 1 *(triglycerides)*	overproduction of VLDL underutilization of VLDL

3.33.) <u>HYPERLIPIDEMIA DRUGS</u>

Diet is the most important factor, improving all types. Drugs are indicated for genetic causes, or if lipid levels cannot be controlled by diet alone.

	MECHANISM OF ACTION / SIDE-EFFECTS	INDICATION
diet	• helps all types of hyperlipidemia • is the only option for type I	all types
niacin	• inhibits lipolysis in fat cells • decreases free fatty acids (decreased VLDL synthesis) ☹ cutaneous flush	type IIB
clofibrate	• activates lipoprotein lipase (increases VLDL utilization) • inhibits cholesterol synthesis • enhances cholesterol excretion in bile ☹ forms gallstones	types III, IV
cholestyramine colestipol	• anion exchanger (binds cholesterol in gut) ☹ interferes with absorption of many drugs[1]	types IIA, IIB
lovastatin	• inhibits HMG-CoA reductase ☹ liver toxicity contraindicated during pregnancy	types IIA, IIB

[1] *don't give at the same time !*

3.34.) PEPTIC ULCERS

H. pylori is the primary cause of peptic ulcer disease, rendering the mucosa susceptible to acids. Eradication of *H. pylori* usually leads to lasting remission.

H₂ blockers	cimetidine	☹ anti-androgenic action
	ranitidine	• more potent, longer acting • no anti-androgenic action
	famotidine	• most potent
prostaglandins	misoprostol	• analog of PGE
proton pump inhibitors	omeprazole	• **drug of choice !**
anti muscarinic	pirenzepine	• reduces acid secretion • less effect on motility • usually combined with others
antacids	Al (OH)₃	☹ may cause constipation
	Mg (OH)₃	☹ may cause diarrhea
mucosa protection	bismuth sucralfate	

> **Eradication of *H. pylori*:**
> metronidazole + tetracycline + bismuth

 Refractory ulcers → suspect Zollinger-Ellison syndrome.
(gastrinoma of pancreas or duodenum)

3.35.) ADRENERGIC DRUGS

A) DIRECT ADRENERGIC DRUGS act directly on adrenergic receptors.

		RECEPTOR ACTION	MAIN INDICATIONS
α-blockers	• phenoxybenzamine • phentolamine • prazosin	α1 , α2, irreversible α1 , α2, reversible α1	• autonomic hyperreflexia • hypertensive crisis • hypertension
α-agonists	• phenylephrine • methoxamine • clonidine	α1 α1 α2 , central action	• nasal decongestant • hypotension • hypertension

β-blockers	• propanolol
	• pindolol
	• metoprolol
	• atenolol
	• labetalol
		β1 , β2
		β1 , β2 , intrinsic act.
		β1
		β1
		β , α
			⎱ hypertension
			   migraine prophylaxis
			   glaucoma

β-agonists	• isoproterenol • metaproterenol, albuterol, terbutaline • dobutamine • dopamine	β1 , β2 β2 β1 D1 > β1	• AV block • bronchospasm • congestive heart failure • shock

B) INDIRECT ADRENERGIC DRUGS modify the amount of norepinephrine at the postsynaptic membrane.

indirect −	• reserpine • guanethidine	depletes neuro- transmitter stores	• hypertension • hypertension
indirect +	• ephedrine • amphetamine	prolongs neuro- transmitter action	• nasal decongestant • narcolepsy, ADHD

3.36.) <u>CHOLINESTERASE INHIBITORS</u>

Acetylcholinesterase splits ACh into acetate and choline and terminates its action. Inhibitors of this enzyme increase the amount of ACh at the neuromuscular junction and parasympathetic nerve endings.

	USE	KEY FEATURES
physostigmine	treatment of M.G.	☹ may cause CNS convulsions
neostigmine	treatment of M.G.	• does not enter CNS • better action on skeletal muscle
edrophonium	diagnosis of M.G.	• shortest duration of action
organophosphates	nerve gas insecticide	• irreversible (highly toxic)

M.G. = myasthenia gravis (autoantibodies against muscle ACh receptor)

Diagnosis of myasthenia gravis (Tensilon test):
Myasthenic crisis: edrophonium improves muscle strength
Cholinergic crisis: edrophonium further reduces muscle strength

---

Organophosphates directly inhibit ACh esterase and slowly form an irreversible complex with the esterase ("aging"). Pralidoxime prevents "aging" and releases active ACh esterase when given early.

3.37.) <u>CHOLINERGIC DRUGS</u>

DIRECT MUSCARINIC DRUGS:

➢ stimulate muscarinic receptors at parasympathetic nerve terminals

	MAIN INDICATIONS	RECEPTOR ACTION
bethanechol	• atonic bladder	muscarinic
pilocarpine [1]	• acute glaucoma	muscarinic
carbachol [1]	• glaucoma • not hydrolyzed by ACh-esterase	muscarinic / nicotinic

[1] *produces miosis (small pupils*
opens outflow (canal of Schlemm) → reduces ocular pressure

Automatic bladder: Spinal cord damage above sacral cord
→ *micturition reflex intact*
→ *but loss of conscious control over reflex*

Atonic bladder: Caused by destruction of sensory nerves
Injury to sacral spinal cord → loss of micturition reflex

Spinal shock: *temporary loss of micturition reflex*

3.38.) ANTI-MUSCARINIC DRUGS

➤ inhibit muscarinic receptors at parasympathetic nerve terminals

	USE
atropine	• anti-spasmodic • mydriasis (large pupils) to facilitate ophthalmologic examination • antidote for organophosphate poisoning
scopolamine	• greater CNS action than atropine for motion sickness

3.39.) ANTI-NICOTINIC DRUGS

➤ inhibit nicotinic receptors at the motor endplates

	ACTIONS / USE
tubocurarine	• blocks nicotinic ACh receptor • muscle relaxant (surgery) ☹ histamine release → bronchospasm hypotension
pancuronium	☺ less histamine release than tubocurarine
succinyl choline	• depolarizing • very short duration of action ☹ post-op muscle pain and stiffness risk of malignant hyperthermia [1]

[1] Ca^{2+} release from SR → muscles generate heat → life threatening!

Be careful with drugs that enhance neuromuscular block:
➤ halothane
➤ aminoglycosides
➤ Ca^{2+} channel blockers

3.40.) ORAL CONTRACEPTIVES

A) USES:

estrogen	• "morning after pill"
progesterone	• "mini pill" • habitual abortion • endometriosis
combination	• oral contraceptive • hormone replacement

B) SIDE-EFFECTS:

Oral contraceptives contain a mixture of estrogen and progesterone. You should adjust the prescription depending on the side-effect your patient experiences:

ESTROGENS ☹	PROGESTERONES ☹
• nausea • vomiting • breast tenderness • skin pigmentation • hypertension • breakthrough bleeding	• weight gain • depression • hirsutism

---

RISKS OF ORAL CONTRACEPTIVES:
- ➢ thromboembolia
- ➢ benign adenoma of the liver
- ➢ vaginal cancer in daughters of mothers who received DES

- ➢ very slight breast cancer or endometrial cancer
  (provided estrogen is combined with progesterone!)

3.41.) STREET DRUGS

HALLUCINOGENS:

	KEY FEATURES
LSD	• acts on 5-HT$_1$ and 5-HT$_2$ receptors

	• activates sympathetic system → arousal
	      tachycardia
	      sweating

	• brilliant color hallucinations (these are blockable by neuroleptics)
	• may trigger schizophreniform psychosis
	• flashbacks
MDMA ("raves")	• popular at dance scene "the raves" • euphoria and confidence • deaths have occurred due to dehydration

 Flashback: *Recurrence of drug effect without the drug.*

OTHERS:

THC (marihuana)	• enhanced sensory activity • impaired mental activity, sleepiness • altered sense of time and self • impaired short term memory • red conjunctivas
phencyclidine ("angel dust")	• reuptake inhibitor • mood elevation, sense of intoxication • bizarre and aggressive behavior

(see 3.45 for amphetamines)

164

3.42.) OPIOIDS

Opioids have the potential to cause strong psychological and physical dependence. Withdrawal (→CNS hyperactivity) is severe, but self-limited and not life-threatening.

A) ENDORPHINS (ENDOGENOUS OPIOID PEPTIDES):

	RECEPTOR	EFFECT
met-enkephalin	mu	• euphoria, dependence • analgesia • respiratory depression
leu-enkephalin	delta	• mood changes
dynorphin	kappa	• analgesia, miosis, sedation

 Morphine (like met-enkephalin) acts on mu receptors.

B) SYNTHETIC OPIOIDS:

Tend to be under-prescribed because of physicians' fear of causing dependence…

	KEY FEATURES
naloxone	• μ, κ, σ antagonist • reverses morphine overdose
pentazocine	• κ, σ agonist / δ, μ antagonist • less effective for severe pain than morphine • less potential for dependence
codeine	• weak analgesic ("as strong as aspirin") • good antitussive • low abuse potential
propoxyphene	**dextro** : analgesic **levo** : antitussive
fentanyl	• 80x analgesic potency of morphine
methadone	• longer duration of action than morphine • used for controlled withdrawal

3.43.) ANTIDEPRESSANTS

Response to antidepressants takes 3-4 weeks. Therapy should continue for several months.
Ask your patient about suicide and offer supportive (not analytic!) psychotherapy.

	MECHANISM OF ACTION	KEY FEATURES
"New Generation" fluoxetine trazodone	• selectively block **serotonin** (5-HT) uptake	• drug of first choice ☺ no anticholinergic side-effects 5-HT1 → antidepressant 5-HT2 → nervousness, insomnia 5 HT3 → nausea, headache
Tricyclic antidepressants amitriptyline amoxapine desipramine etc.	• block neurotransmitter uptake (NE, serotonin, dopamine) • block receptors (m, α, serotonin, histamine)	• slow onset of action • inconsistent bioavailability ☹ **anticholinergic side-effects:** - blurred vision, dry mouth - constipation - urinary retention
MAO inhibitors	• increases amount of transmitter stored	• use when other drugs have failed • have stimulant properties • caveat: tyramine

Tyramine (cheese, beer, red wine) normally is inactivated by MAO in gut. When it gets into the circulation → hypertensive crisis!

3.44.) LITHIUM
Therapeutic range: 0.5-1 mEq/L

Lithium is a "mood-stabilizer", effective for bipolar disorder and isolated manic episodes. Treatment of a manic episode should continue for at least 6 months. Because of its very low therapeutic index you must carefully monitor your patients for side-effects:

key features	⊗ extremely low therapeutic index • excreted by kidneys
indications	• to treat manic episodes • to stabilize mood (prevents both manic and depressive episodes)
"normal" side-effects	• mild nausea • thirst
early intoxication 1.5 - 2 mEq/L	• abdominal pain, vomiting • hand tremor • ataxia, nystagmus • slurred speech
severe intoxication > 2 mEq/L	• persistent vomiting • blurred vision • hyperactive tendon reflexes • convulsions, coma, death

3.45.) CNS STIMULANTS

CNS stimulants cause psychological dependence (most profound for cocaine). Physical dependence is less with these drugs.

	KEY FEATURES
methylxanthines caffeine, theophylline	**low dose:** increased alertness **high dose:** anxiety, tremors • smooth muscle relaxation • weak diuretic • enhanced acid secretion in stomach
nicotine	**low dose:** ganglion stimulating, BP ↑ **high dose:** ganglion blockade, BP ↓
cocaine	• reuptake inhibitor • local anesthetic and vasoconstrictor • euphoria, hallucinations delusions, paranoia • cardiac arrhythmias
crack cocaine	• quicker effect, more intense "high"
amphetamines	• release of stored catecholamines • effects like cocaine • euphoria lasts longer than cocaine • no tolerance to CNS toxicity
methamphetamines	• common form of amphetamine abuse in US • can be smoked as "ice"

Dextroamphetamine: *- strong appetite suppressant*
- euphoria, risk of dependence
- not recommended for weight loss!

Attention-Deficit-Hyperactivity-Disorder:
Children with ADHD have a "paradoxical" reaction
to amphetamines: It calms them down!

3.46.) ANXIOLYTIC DRUGS

Anxiety is often a/w medical or psychiatric problems. Best response to anxiolytics occurs in relatively acute anxiety reactions. Chronic use may lead to dependence.

		KEY FEATURES
benzodiazepines	diazepam	• long acting • for status epilepticus
	chlordiazepoxide	• long acting • for alcohol withdrawal
	lorazepam, triazolam	• rapid elimination (short half life) → ☹ severe withdrawal symptoms
others	buspirone	• acts on 5-HT1A receptors • slow onset of action • less sedation • less dependence

 Abrupt withdrawal may cause delirium and seizures!

3.47.) HYPNOTIC DRUGS

These drugs cause widespread depression of CNS → risk of respiratory depression
(suicidal potential)

		KEY FEATURES
barbiturates	phenobarbital	• long acting, for seizure disorder
	thiopental	• short acting, for anesthesia
others	chloral hydrate	• recommended for children ☹ causes epigastric pain
	meprobamate	• less sedation, better anxiolytic

3.48.) ANTIHISTAMINES

H1 receptors	• nasal and bronchial secretions • constrict bronchial smooth muscle → asthma • dilate skin capillaries → redness, wheals, itch
H2 receptors	• acid secretion in stomach

Antihistamines are the drug of choice for allergic rhinitis and urticaria.
The major side-effect is sedation:

	KEY FEATURES
diphenhydramine	indications: • allergic rhinitis • urticaria • not effective in asthma ☹ sedation
carbinoxamine	☺ less drowsiness than diphenhydramine
trimeprazine (phenothiazine)	• long half life • good antipruritic
terfenadine, astemizole	• non-sedating antihistamines

For motion sickness and nausea:
• diphenhydramine (antihistamine)
• meclizine (antihistamine)
• scopolamine (phenothiazine)

3.49.) ANESTHETICS

The minimum alveolar concentration (MAC) is the gas concentration needed to prevent movement of patients subjected to painful stimuli. MAC depends on the blood/gas partition (solubility). If the partition coefficient is high, a low alveolar concentration is sufficient but onset and termination of anesthesia will be slow.

> **MAC :** N_2O > enflurane > halothane
>
> **onset :** N_2O > enflurane > halothane
> fastest.....................slowest

A) INHALATION:

	KEY FEATURES
halothane	• lacks analgesic potency ☹ hepatotoxic for adults cardiac arrhythmias malignant hyperthermia
enflurane	• excreted by kidney rather than liver
isoflurane	• does not induce arrhythmias • lower toxicity
N_2O (nitrous oxide)	• not potent • does not depress respiration • safe

B) I.V.:

thiopental	• ultrashort barbiturate • not analgesic
ketamine	• dissociative anesthesia (patient appears awake but is unaware of pain) ☹ postoperative hallucinations

> ➢ balanced anesthesia: thiopental + fentanyl + tubocurarine + N_2O
> ➢ neurolept anesthesia: droperidol + fentanyl + N_2O

3.50.) PARKINSON'S DISEASE

Parkinson's is due to loss of dopaminergic substantia nigra neurons which project to the basal ganglia. This results in a neurotransmitter imbalance. Symptoms can be improved by either increasing dopamine or decreasing acetylcholine in the basal ganglia:

dopaminergic	**levodopa**	• CNS permeable dopamine • (**carbidopa** inhibits peripheral decarboxylase) ☹ nausea, vomiting dyskinesia psychic disturbances
	bromocriptine	• direct dopamine agonist
	deprenyl	• inhibits MAO-B (dopamine selective)
	amantadine	• enhances dopamine metabolism
anticholinergic	**benztropine** **biperiden**	☹ dry mouth mydriasis tachycardia constipation urinary retention

> <u>Early disease:</u>
> If symptoms are mild, no drugs may be necessary
> Otherwise start with anticholinergics or amantadine
>
> <u>Fully developed disease:</u>
> Levodopa plus Carbidopa
>
> <u>Late stage:</u>
> "wearing off" of drug effect
> "on-off" phenomenon
> may need to reduce levodopa if dyskinesias develop
> may need to combine several drugs

3.51.) NEUROLEPTICS

Antipsychotic drugs (neuroleptics) are used to treat schizophrenia. They have a high affinity for dopamine D2 receptors. Their Parkinson-like side-effects are due to block of dopamine receptors in the basal ganglia.

		KEY FEATURES
phenothiazines	chlorpromazine	☹ anticholinergic side effects arrhythmias rarely used
	fluphenazine	• long acting • for outpatients
butyrophenones	haloperidol	☹ extrapyramidal side effects fewer anticholinergic side effects
	droperidol	• for neurolept anesthesia
other	clozapine	☹ bone marrow suppression fewer extrapyramidal side effects

---

☹ **DYSKINESIAS CAUSED BY NEUROLEPTICS:**
- **Acute dystonia** occurs within hours of administration.
- torticollis, jaw dislocation, tongue protrusion
  usually disappears (tolerance)

- **Parkinsonism** occurs within weeks to months of treatment.
- muscle stiffness, cogwheel rigidity, shuffling, drooling
  usually disappears (tolerance)

- **Tardive dyskinesia** occurs after many months of treatment.
- choreoathetosis, tongue protrusion, lateral movements of jaw
  may be irreversible!

3.52.) ANTIEPILEPTIC DRUGS

Seizures are due to sudden abnormal electrical activity in the cortex. It may be focal or spread and cause generalized convulsions. Antiepileptic drugs reduce neuronal excitability and prolong the refractory period of the action potentials.

DISORDER	DRUG OF CHOICE
generalized tonic-clonic (grand mal)	phenytoin, carbamazepine
partial focal	phenytoin, carbamazepine
absence seizures (petit mal)	ethosuximide
myoclonic	valproic acid, clonazepam
febrile seizures (children)	phenobarbital
status epilepticus [1]	diazepam I.V.

[1] *Medical emergency! Keep airways open!*

3.53.) ANTIEMETIC DRUGS

Antiemetics act on the chemoreceptor trigger zone of the brain stem (vomiting center). For unknown reasons some drugs work better than others depending on the clinical situation:

CLINICAL SITUATION	DRUG OF CHOICE
motion sickness	• scopolamine, • diphenhydramine
vertigo	• meclizine
chemotherapy	• metoclopramide
radiation therapy	• domperidone

3.54.) LAXATIVES

bulk forming [1] (stool softeners)	• fibers (fruit, vegetable) • methyl cellulose • psyllium seeds
irritants (increased intestinal motility)	• senna • castor oil
nonabsorbable salines [1] (increased osmotic pressure)	• magnesium salts
lubricants (to protect hemorrhoids)	• mineral oil

[1] *take with plenty of water*

Abuse of laxatives → *intestinal potassium loss* → *hypokalemia* → *decreased intestinal motility* → *increased "need" for laxatives*

BIOCHEMISTRY

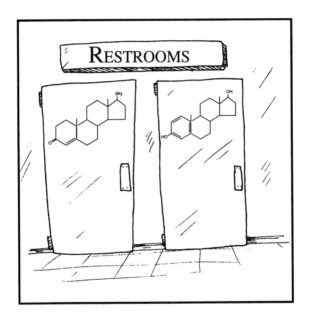

4.1.) <u>ENZYME KINETICS</u>

The Lineweaver-Burke plot is a convenient way to show the relationship between [substrate] concentration and rate of reaction (V):

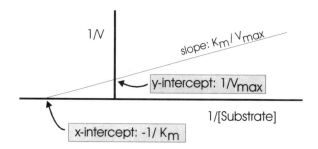

V_{max}: *Maximal rate of reaction when enzyme is saturated with substrate.*

K_m: *Substrate concentration at which reaction rate is half of its maximal value.*
High K_m = low affinity
Low K_m = high affinity

<u>COMPETITIVE INHIBITOR</u>: (binds at same site as substrate)

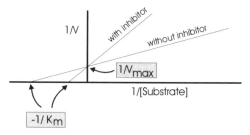

<u>NONCOMPETITIVE INHIBITOR</u>: (binds at different site from substrate)

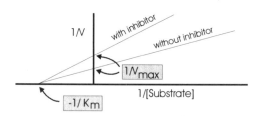

4.2.) <u>AMINO ACIDS</u>

Only 20 amino acids are commonly found in mammalian cells. Amino acids have an amino and a carboxyl group, forming peptide bonds with each other:

$$A_1 - COO^- + \ ^+H_3N - A_2 \ \rightarrow \ A_1 - \underset{O}{\overset{H}{\underset{\|}{C} - N}} - A_2$$

acidic	aspartate, glutamate
basic	histidine, lysine, arginine
essential	valine, leucin, isoleucine tryptophan, phenylalanine, methionine lysine, arginine histidine, threonine
strictly ketogenic	leucine, lysine
keto- and glucogenic	isoleucine, threonine tryptophan, phenylalanine

Glucogenic: if carbon skeleton can be converted to glucose.
Ketogenic: if carbon skeleton can be converted to acetyl CoA.

trypsin cleaves at	$^+NH_3$ - [Arg or Lys] ✓ - [any] - COO^-
chymotrypsin cleaves at	$^+NH_3$ - [Phe, Tyr, Trp or Leu] ✓ - [any] - COO^-

179

4.3.) <u>AMINO ACID PRECURSORS</u>

Amino acids are not only the building blocks of proteins, they are also used to form a number of biologically active molecules:

	PRODUCTS:
tyrosine	• dopa, dopamine • norepinephrine, epinephrine • T3, T4 (thyroxin) • melanin
tryptophan	• 5-HT (serotonin) • melatonin • niacin
glutamate	• GABA
glycine	• porphyrin, heme • creatine (glycine plus + arginine)
histidine	• histamine

4.4.) AMINO ACID DISORDERS

Inborn errors of metabolism prevent proper catabolism of amino acids. Most clinical symptoms are due to accumulation of metabolites.

A) ENZYMES:

	DEFECT	SIGNS & SYMPTOMS
albinism	tyrosinase	• unpigmented skin, eyes
phenylketonuria	phenylalanine hydroxylase	• mental retardation • hypopigmentation • musty odor
alkaptonuria	homogentisate oxidase	• arthritis (ochronosis) • urine darkens
maple syrup	branched chain decarboxylase	• hyperreflexia • sweet odor urine
homocystinuria	cystathionine synthetase	• mental retardation • lens dislocation

B) TRANSPORTERS: (kidneys and intestinal epithelium)

	DEFECT	SIGNS & SYMPTOMS
cystinuria	dibasic amino acid transporter [1]	• urinary cystine stones
Hartnup disease	neutral amino acid transporter [1]	tryptophan deficiency ↓ niacin deficiency ↓ pellagra

> **PELLAGRA** (Hartnup disease or dietary niacin deficiency):
> "3 Ds": Dermatitis,   Dementia,   Diarrhea

4.5.) <u>ENZYME DEFECTS</u>

<u>ALBINISM</u>: defective tyrosinase in melanocytes

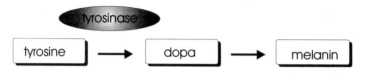

Nerve cell tyrosinase is intact.
(patients can still make epinephrine and norepinephrine).

<u>PHENYLKETONURIA</u>: defective phenylalanine hydroxylase

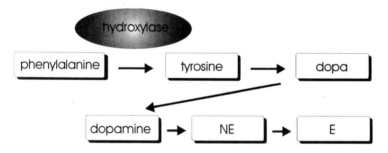

Tyrosine become an essential amino acid in patients with phenylketonuria.

<u>ALKAPTONURIA</u>: defective homogentisate oxidase

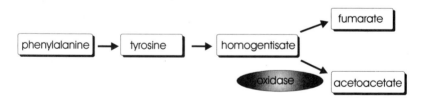

MAPLE SYRUP DISEASE: defective branched chain decarboxylase

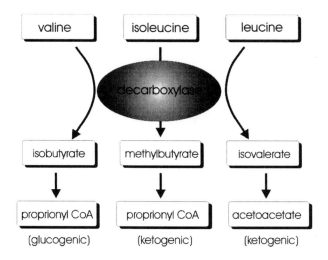

Accumulation of branched chain keto acids gives urine a sweet odor.

HOMOCYSTINURIA: defective cystathione synthase

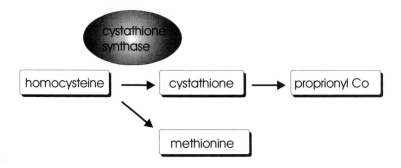

homocysteine + homocysteine → homocystine (in urine)

4.6.) <u>MONOSACCHARIDES</u>

Monosaccharides are simple sugars that are classified by the number of C atoms: pentose=5, hexose = 6. There are several isomers of each sugar (i.e. same chemical formula, different configuration):

<u>EPIMERS OF GLUCOSE:</u>

αD-glucose	mannose	galactose
β CHO α	CHO	CHO
2- OH	OH - 2	2- OH
OH - 3	OH - 3	OH - 3
4-OH	4-OH	OH - 4
L 5-OH D	5-OH	5-OH
CH_2OH	CH_2OH	CH_2OH

pyranose	• ring with <u>5 carbons + 1 oxygen</u> *(example: glucose)*
furanose	• ring with <u>4 carbons + 1 oxygen</u> *(example: fructose)*
anomeric carbon	• C atom that has <u>4 different ligands</u> *(for sugars this refers to the C1 in ring form)*
epimers	• **isomers that differ in only <u>one</u> carbon** *(example: glucose and galactose)*
enantiomers	• mirror image (i.e. flipped at all anomeric C atoms)
reducing sugars	• oxygen on C1 atom is available for redox reaction • glucose, galactose and fructose are reducing sugars • sucrose is a non-reducing sugar

4.7.) <u>HEXOSE KINASES</u>

These enzymes phosphorylate glucose to glucose-6-phosphate, which cannot get out of the cell. Glucokinase of the liver has a lower affinity, removing glucose when blood concentrations are high.

	hexokinase	glucokinase
organs	many	liver
substrate specificity	many hexoses	many hexoses
affinity	**high**	low
V_{max} ("capacity")	low	**high**
inhibited by glucose-6 phosphate	yes	no

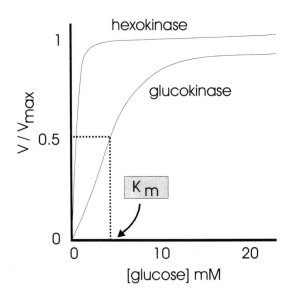

4.8.) <u>SACCHARIDES</u>

Saccharides are carbohydrates composed of several monosaccharides.

> **α-bond:** carbon 1 is in α position (down)
> **β-bond:** carbon 1 is in β position (up)

A) <u>DISACCHARIDES</u>:

	COMPOSITION	BOND
maltose (beer)	glucose + glucose	α1 - 4
lactose (milk)	galactose + glucose	β1 - 4
sucrose (table sugar)	glucose + fructose	α1 - β2

B) <u>POLYSACCHARIDES</u>:

	composition	bonds
glycogen, starch	many glucoses	α1 - 4 (chains) α1 - 6 (branch points)
cellulose	many glucoses	β1 - 4

The β1- 4 bond cannot be hydrolyzed by humans. (Cellulose is indigestible.)

4.9.) <u>SACCHARIDE DISORDERS</u>

Inborn errors of metabolism that prevent digestion or catabolism of saccharides. Clinical symptoms are mostly due to accumulation of metabolites.

	ENZYME DEFECT	SIGNS & SYMPTOMS
fructosuria	fructokinase	• benign • asymptomatic
fructose intolerance	aldolase B	• hypoglycemia • liver failure
galactosemia	uridyltransferase	• cataracts • mental retardation
lactose intolerance	lactase (usually acquired)	• diarrhea

 Diarrhea of any cause can result in temporary lactase deficiency. (Don't drink milk if you have diarrhea!)

4.10.) <u>ENZYME DEFECTS</u>

<u>FRUCTOSE INTOLERANCE</u>: defective fructokinase or aldolase-B

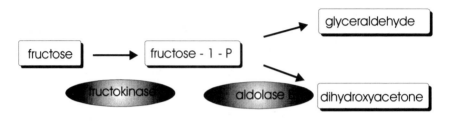

Fructosuria (defective fructokinase): Fructose is harmless.

Fructose intolerance (defective aldolase): Fructose-1-P accumulates in liver and inhibits glycogenolysis and gluconeogenesis → severe hypoglycemia.

<u>GALACTOSEMIA</u>: defective uridyltransferase

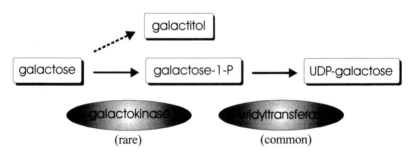

Many States in the US require newborn screening for this disease because failure to treat results in early mental retardation.

4.11.) <u>GLYCOGEN STORAGE DISEASES</u>

Glucose-6-phosphate cannot cross cell membranes. In Von Gierke disease, glucose-6-phosphate remains trapped inside the liver cells and inhibits glycogen breakdown.

Some glycogen is continuously degraded by lysosomal α-glucosidase. Deficiency results in glycogen accumulation in all organs.

Glycogen phosphorylase cleaves the α1-4 bond and releases glucose-1-phosphate.

	ENZYME DEFECT	ORGANS AFFECTED
Type I Von Gierke	glucose-6-phosphatase	• liver and kidneys enlarged • fasting hypoglycemia • acidosis • failure to thrive
Type II Pompe	α-glucosidase (lysosomes)	• affects all organs • muscle hypotonia • cardiac failure • death before age 2
Type V McArdle	skeletal muscle 　　　glycogen phosphorylase	• exercise: muscle pain/cramps • progressive muscle weakness

 Skeletal muscle cells don't have glucose-6-phosphatase (unlike the liver, muscle cells do not release glucose into the circulation).

4.12.) <u>ENZYME DEFECTS</u>

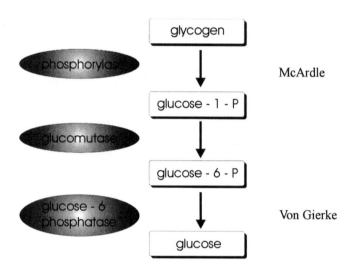

The enzyme defect in Type II (Pompe) involves a lysosomal enzyme of an alternate pathway of glycogen breakdown.

4.13.) GLYCOSAMINOGLYCANS
(mucopolysaccharides)

Long, unbranched polysaccharides composed of repeating disaccharides.
One of the disaccharides is a hexosamine (often N-acetyl-glucosamine).
They can bind large amounts of water ($\rightarrow$ gel) and provide lubrication.

> ## Common glycosaminoglycans:
> o hyaluronic acid
> o heparin
> o keratan sulfate
> o chondroitin sulfate
> o dermatan sulfate

SOME MUCOPOLYSACCHARIDOSES:

	ENZYME DEFECT	SIGNS & SYMPTOMS
Hurler	α-L Iduronidase [1]	• cornea clouding • mental retardation
Scheie	α-L Iduronidase [1]	• cornea clouding • normal intelligence
Hunter	Iduronate sulfatase	• no clouding • mental retardation

[1] *same enzyme, different mutations*

PROTEOGLYCANS:
• Proteoglycans have a protein core to which numerous side chains of glycosaminoglycans attach.
• Major functions: Lubricants, extracellular matrix, molecular "sieve".

4.14.) <u>FATTY ACIDS</u>

Fatty acids are rich in energy and needed for many physiological processes. Linoleic and arachidonic acid are "essential", i.e. cannot be synthesized by human cells. Infants should NOT be fed skim-milk formulas!

<u>SATURATED</u>:

	STRUCTURE	FEATURES
palmitic acid	16:0	• product of human fatty acid synthesis
stearic acid	18:0	

<u>MONOUNSATURATED</u>: (have one C=C double bound)

palmitoleic acid	16:1(9)	
oleic acid	18:1(9)	

<u>POLYUNSATURATED</u>: (have several C=C double bounds)

linoleic acid	18:2(9,12)	• plant oils
linolenic acid	18:3(9,12,15)	
arachidonic acid	20:4(5,8,11,14)	• precursor of prostaglandins

Example: 18:1(9): 18 carbons, 1 double bond at position 9

- o Peripheral atherosclerosis correlates with saturated fat intake.
- o Margarine (hydrogenated vegetable oils = <u>trans</u> fatty acids) is similarly harmful.

4.15.) <u>BILE ACIDS</u>

Bile acids are amphipathic (have both polar and unpolar parts) allowing them to emulsify otherwise insoluble lipids. If bile contains more cholesterol than what can be solubilized by bile acids and phospholipids, it will crystallize and form stones.

	BILE ACIDS	FEATURES
primary	• cholic acid • chenodeoxycholic acid	• derived from cholesterol
secondary	• deoxycholic acid • lithocholic acid	• produced from primary conjugated bile salts by intestinal bacteria • less soluble → excreted
conjugate	• glycocholic acid (cholic acid + glycine) • taurocholic acid (cholic acid + taurine)	• ionized at physiologic pH • form micelles with dietary fats

 >95% of bile salts are reabsorbed in the ileum. ("Enterohepatic circulation")

4.16.) <u>PHOSPHOLIPIDS</u>

<u>TRIGLYCERIDES</u>   <u>GLYCERO-PHOSPHOLIPIDS</u>

<u>CERAMIDE</u>   <u>SPHINGO-PHOSPHOLIPIDS</u>

<u>CEREBROSIDES</u>   <u>GANGLIOSIDES</u>

A) GLYCERO-PHOSPHOLIPIDS:
(spontaneously form lipid bilayers → cell membranes)

phosphatidyl choline (= lecithin)	phosphatidic acid + choline
phosphatidyl ethanolamine	phosphatidic acid + ethanolamine
phosphatidyl serine	phosphatidic acid + serine
phosphatidyl inositol	phosphatidic acid + inositol
cardiolipin	2x phosphatidic acid + glycerine

= "head"

B) SPHINGO-PHOSPHOLIPIDS:

ceramide	sphingosine + fatty acid
sphingomyelin	ceramide + choline

4.17.) GLYCOLIPIDS

cerebroside	ceramide + mono saccharide
globoside	ceramide + oligosaccharide
ganglioside	ceramide + oligosaccharide + NANA

4.18.) SPHINGOLIPIDOSES

Inborn errors of metabolism that prevent catabolism of sphingolipids. Clinical symptoms are due to accumulation of metabolites.

		ACCUMULATE/ENZYME	SIGNS & SYMPTOMS
Niemann-Pick	A	sphingomyelin/ sphingomyelinase	• liver and spleen enlargement • foamy cells
Gaucher	A	glucocerebrosides/ β-glucosidase	• liver and spleen enlargement • osteoporosis • Ashkenazi Jews
Krabbe	A	galactocerebrosides/ β-galactosidase	• blindness, deafness • convulsions • globoid cells
metachromatic leukodystrophy	A	sulfatides/ arylsulfatase	• progressive paralysis
Fabry	X	globosides/ α-galactosidase	• reddish-purple skin rash • kidney/heart failure • angiokeratoma
Tay-Sachs	A	gangliosides/ hexosaminidase	• blindness • cherry red macula • Ashkenazi Jews

A = Autosomal recessive
X = X-linked recessive

4.19.) ENZYME DEFECTS

GALACTOSE: defective arylsulfatase or β-galactosidase

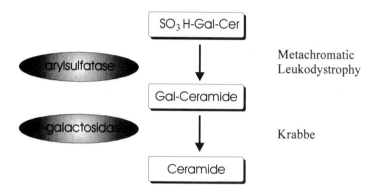

SO$_3$H-Gal-Cer

Metachromatic
Leukodystrophy

Gal-Ceramide

Krabbe

Ceramide

GLUCOSE: defective β-glucosidase

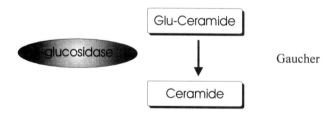

Glu-Ceramide

Gaucher

Ceramide

4.20.) <u>PORPHYRIAS</u>

Heme is an iron-containing derivative of porphyrin. Porphyrias are due to defects in heme biosynthesis and as a result precursors of heme accumulate.

	ACCUMULATE	PHOTO-SENSITIVITY	OTHER SIGNS
acute intermittent	porphobilinogen [1]	no	• abdominal pain
cutanea tarda	uroporphyrinogen	yes	
coproporphyria	coproporphyrinogen	yes	• abdominal pain
lead poisoning	δ-ALA protoporphyrin	no	• anemia *microcytic, hypochrome* *basophil stippling*

[1] precipitated by dieting, steroids, sulfonamides and many other drugs.

<u>MECHANISM OF PHOTOSENSITIVITY:</u>

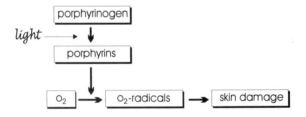

4.21.) <u>ENZYME DEFECTS</u>

Heme is used in hemoglobin, myoglobin and cytochromes and synthesized from δ-aminolevulinic acid (glycine + succinyl CoA):

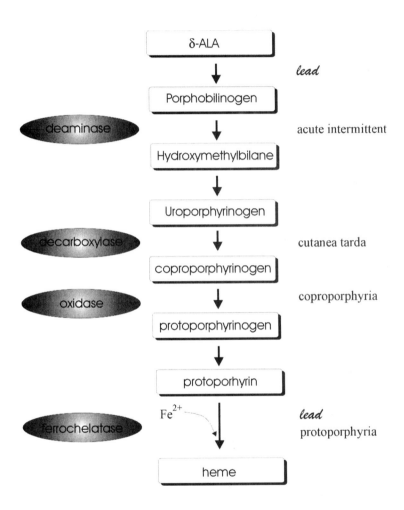

4.22.) PREFERRED NUTRIENTS

The heart is completely aerobic. In contrast, skeletal muscles can function anaerobically for some time. After a prolonged fast, metabolism adapts to preserve amino acids:

	NORMAL	PROLONGED FAST
brain	• glucose	• ketone bodies • glucose
muscle	• **rest:** fatty acids • **exercise:** glucose	• fatty acids
heart ("takes anything")	• fatty acids • ketone bodies • lactate • glucose	• fatty acids • ketone bodies • lactate • glucose
erythrocytes	• glucose	• glucose

The heart is completely aerobic. In contrast, skeletal muscles can function anaerobically for some time.

FASTING:
o The brain and red blood cells always need glucose.
o The liver maintains glucose levels by a) glycogenolysis
                                           b) gluconeogenesis

o Substrates for liver gluconeogenesis: Muscle, RBCs: → lactate
                                           Fat cells: triglycerides → glycerol

o Production of ketones by liver: Triglycerides → fatty acids → ketones

4.23.) <u>VITAMINS</u>

Vitamins are essential nutrients that cannot be synthesized by human cells. Deficiencies are most common in poverty and chronic alcohol abuse.

	FUNCTION	SIGNS OF DEFICIENCY
A	part of rhodopsin	• night blindness (retinal) • growth retardation (retinoic acid)
D	• GI tract: Ca^{2+} absorption • bone : supports PTH	• rickets, osteomalacia
E	• antioxidant	• ataxia
K	• carboxylation of • glutamate	• bleeding disorder (II, VII, IX, X)
C	• hydroxylation of • proline and lysine	• scurvy
B1 (thiamin)	• decarboxylations	• beriberi
B2 (riboflavin)	• flavins (FMN etc.)	• glossitis, cheilosis
B6 (pyridoxine)	• transaminations • deaminations	• anemia (microcytic) • neuropathy
B12	• methionine synthesis • odd carbon fatty acid • degradation	• anemia (macrocytic) • neuropathy • D. Latum (worm infestation)
niacin	• NAD^+, $NADP^+$	• pellagra • (=diarrhea, dementia, dermatitis)
pantothenate	• Coenzyme A	• headache, nausea
biotin	• carboxylations	• seborrheic dermatitis • nervous disorders • avidin (raw egg white) binds biotin
folic acid	• one carbon metabolism	• anemia (macrocytic) • glossitis, colitis

4.24.) <u>ATP EQUIVALENTS</u>

Fat (9 kcal/g) is more rich in energy than protein (4 kcal/g) or sugar (4 kcal/g). Here is why:

	YIELD	EXPLANATION
$FADH_2$	2	
NADH	3	
acetyl CoA	12.	acetyl CoA $\rightarrow$ 2 CO_2 3 NADH + $FADH_2$ + GTP
pyruvate	15	pyruvate $\rightarrow$ acetyl CoA + NADH
glycolysis (anaerobe)	2.	glucose $\rightarrow$ lactate 4 ATP minus 2 ATP [1]
glycolysis (aerobe)	8	glucose $\rightarrow$ pyruvate (4 ATP minus 2 ATP) + 2 NADH
glucose (complete oxidation)	38	glucose $\rightarrow$ 6 CO_2 8 + 2x15 (pyruvate)
fatty acid (e.g. 16:0)	129	
gluconeogenesis (from pyruvate)	-12	
urea synthesis	-4	

[1] 2 ATP required for hexokinase and fructokinase reactions

Glycerophosphate shuttle (yields 2 ATP per NADH)
Reducing equivalents are transferred from cytosolic NADH to mitochondrial $FADH_2$.

Malate shuttle (yields 3 ATP per NADH)
Reducing equivalents are transferred from cytosolic NADH to mitochondrial NADH.

4.25.) KEY ENZYMES - SUGARS

Most metabolic pathways are regulated by one or two "key enzymes" which can be allosterically activated or inhibited. Sometimes enzyme activity is dependent on phosphorylation.

CARBOHYDRATE METABOLISM:

	ENZYME	ALLOSTERIC INHIBITORS	ALLOSTERIC ACTIVATORS	EFFECT OF PHOSPHORYLATION
glycolysis	phosphofructokinase 1	ATP citrate	AMP fructose 2,6 -dp	inhibits
	phosphofructokinase 2			
gluconeogenesis	fructosediphosphatase 1	AMP fructose 2,6 -dp	ATP citrate	
	fructosediphosphatase 2			activates
glycogenolysis	glycogenphosphorylase			activates
glycogen synthesis	glycogen synthetase			inhibits
pentose phosphate shunt	glucose-6-phosphate dehydrogenase	NADPH		

4.26.) KEY ENZYMES - FATS

FAT METABOLISM:

	ENZYME	ALLOSTERIC INHIBITORS	ALLOSTERIC ACTIVATORS	EFFECT OF PHOSPHORYLATION
lipolysis	carnitine acyltransferase	malonyl CoA		
fat mobilization	hormone sensitive lipase			activates
lipid synthesis	acetyl-CoA carboxylase		citrate	inhibits
cholesterol synthesis	HMG CoA reductase		cholesterol	inhibits

4.27.) KEY ENZYMES - OTHERS

OTHER PATHWAYS:

	ENZYME	ALLOSTERIC INHIBITORS	EFFECT OF PHOSPHORYLATION
ketone body synthesis	HMG CoA synthase		
purine synthesis	amidotransferase	AMP GMP IMP	
citric acid cycle	pyruvate dehydrogenase	Acetyl CoA ATP NADH	inhibits

- : allosteric inhibitor

4.28.) STEROIDS

Steroid hormones are made from cholesterol:

CLASS	EXAMPLE	NUMBER OF C-ATOMS
sterols	cholesterol	27
bile acids	glycocholate taurocholate	24
glucocorticoids	cortisol	21
mineralocorticoids	aldosterone	21
gestagens	progesterone	21
androgens	testosterone * androstenedione DHEAS	19
estrogens	estradiol * estriol	18

* most potent

<u>17-ketosteroids</u> (dehydroandrosterone and androstenedione) ↑
- 11-hydroxylase deficiency
- 21-hydroxylase deficiency
- Cushing's syndrome
- androgen producing adrenal or gonadal tumors

<u>17-hydroxysteroids</u> (cortisol metabolites) ↑
- 11-hydroxylase deficiency
- Cushing's syndrome

4.29.) <u>ADRENAL GLAND</u>

Steroid synthesis always follows the same scheme, but different tissues have
different sets of enzymes, resulting in a different product:

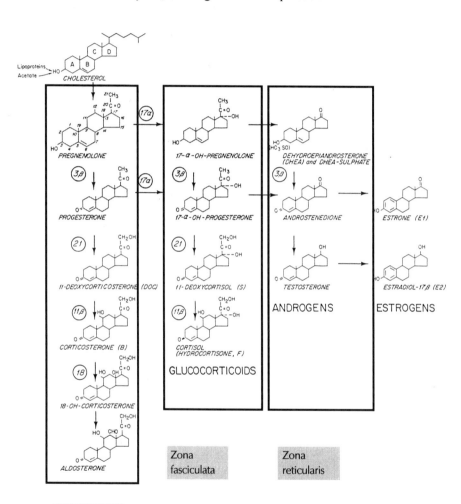

4.30.) <u>TESTIS (Leydig Cells)</u>

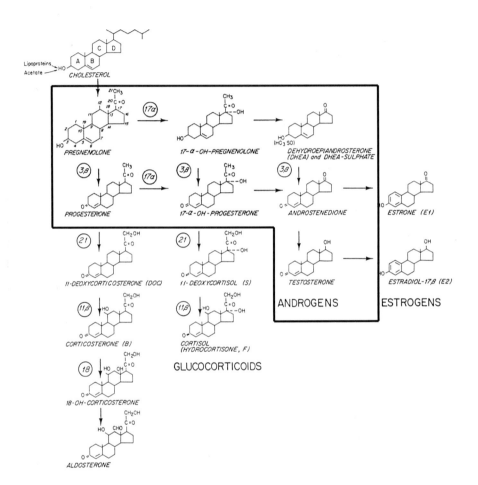

ANDROGENS   ESTROGENS

GLUCOCORTICOIDS

4.31.) <u>PERIPHERAL METABOLISM</u>

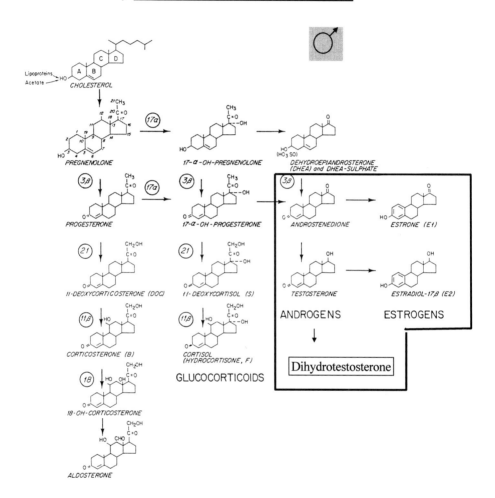

GLUCOCORTICOIDS

ANDROGENS   ESTROGENS

Dihydrotestosterone

4.32.) <u>OVARY (Theca Cells)</u>

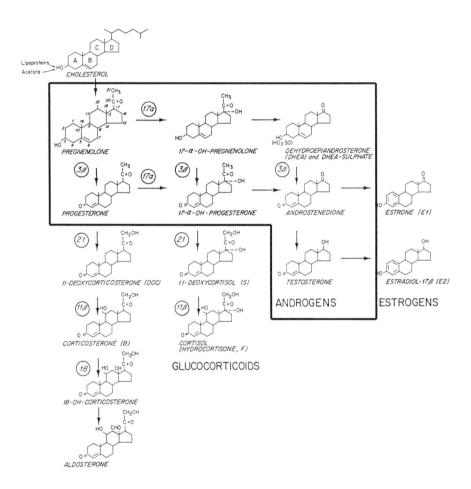

GLUCOCORTICOIDS

4.33.) <u>OVARY (Granulosa Cells)</u>

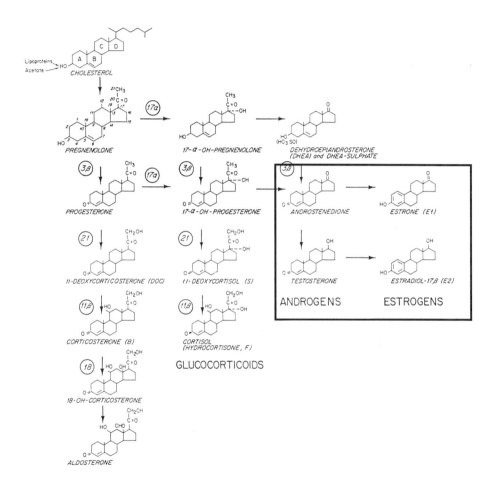

4.34.) <u>PERIPHERAL METABOLISM</u>

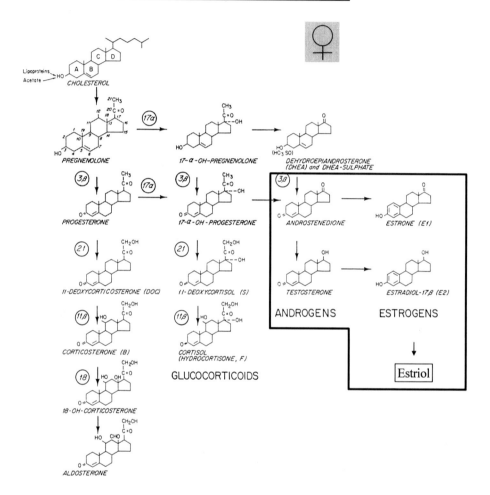

CHOLESTEROL

Lipoproteins
Acetate

PREGNENOLONE

17-α-OH-PREGNENOLONE

DEHYDROEPIANDROSTERONE
(DHEA) and DHEA-SULPHATE

PROGESTERONE

17-α-OH-PROGESTERONE

ANDROSTENEDIONE

ESTRONE (E1)

11-DEOXYCORTICOSTERONE (DOC)

11-DEOXYCORTISOL (S)

TESTOSTERONE

ESTRADIOL-17,β (E2)

CORTICOSTERONE (B)

CORTISOL
(HYDROCORTISONE, F)

ANDROGENS

ESTROGENS

18-OH-CORTICOSTERONE

GLUCOCORTICOIDS

Estriol

ALDOSTERONE

4.35.) <u>CORPUS LUTEUM</u>

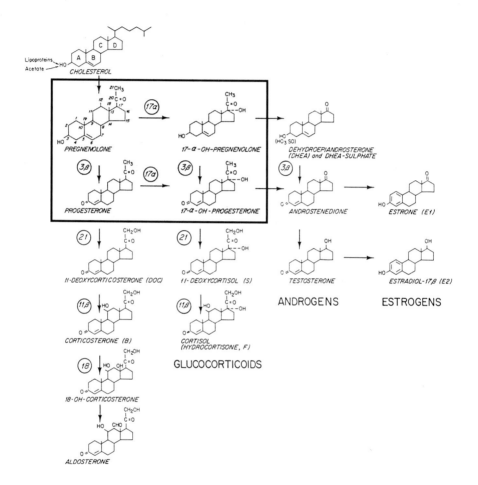

4.36.) 17-α-HYDROXYLASE DEFICIENCY

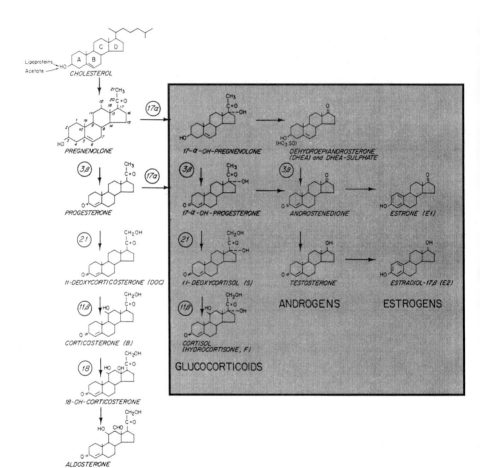

Male :	ambiguous genitalia
Female :	primary amenorrhea at puberty

4.37.) 21-α-HYDROXYLASE DEFICIENCY

most common defect of
corticoid synthesis (95%)

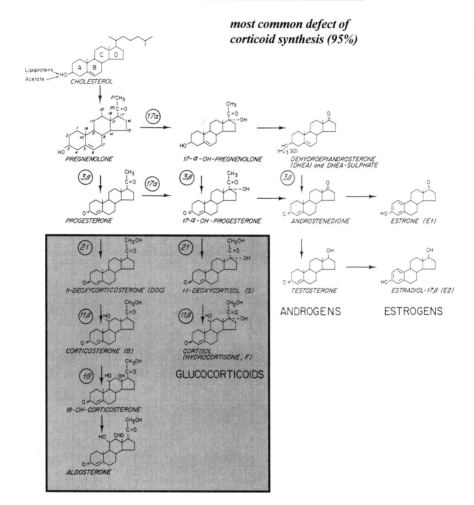

Male :	precocious puberty (DHEA↑)
Female :	ambiguous genitalia (DHEA↑)
Salt wasting:	50-60% of patients (lack of aldosterone)

4.38.) <u>11-β-HYDROXYLASE</u>

Male :	precocious puberty (androgens↑)
Female :	ambiguous genitalia (androgens↑)
Salt retention:	hypertension, hypokalemia
	(deoxycorticosterone has mineralocorticoid action)

4.39.) ENDOCRINE CONTROL OF METABOLISM

	fat	sugar	proteins
insulin	(A) • synthesis	(A) • uptake (M,F) • glycolysis (L,M) • glycogen synthesis (L,M)	(A) • synthesis
glucagon	(C) • lysis	(C) • gluconeogenesis (L) • glycogenolysis (L)	(C) • increases uptake of AA in liver for gluconeogenesis
growth hormone	(C) • lysis	(C) • gluconeogenesis (L)	(A) • synthesis
cortisol	(C) • lysis • redistribution	(A) • inhibits uptake (M,F) • gluconeogenesis (L) • glycogen synthesis (L,M)	(C) • degradation
epinephrine	(C) • lysis	(C) • increases uptake (M) • glycolysis (M) • gluconeogenesis (L) • glycogenolysis (L,M)	-

(A) anabolic   (C) catabolic   M: Muscle   L: Liver   F: Fat

A Insulin has a general anabolic action

A GH promotes synthesis of protein at the expense fat and sugars.

A Cortisol increases blood sugar levels and build-up of glycogen stores at the expense of fat and protein

4.40.) <u>NUCLEOTIDES</u>

Nucleosides are purines or pyrimidines linked to a pentose sugar.
Nucleotides are phosphates (mono-, di- or ti-) of the nucleoside.

BASE	NUCLEOSIDE	NUCLEOTIDE
PURINES:		
• adenine	• adenosine	• adenylate (AMP)
• guanine	• guanosine	• guanylate (GMP)
PYRIMIDINES:		
• uracil	• uridine	• uridylate (UMP)
• cytosine	• cytidine	• cytidylate (CMP)
• thymine	• deoxythymidine	• deoxythymidylate (dTMP)

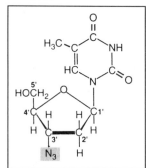

Thymidine: AZT:

*AZT (Zidovudine) can be incorporated into DNA by viral
reverse transcriptase. Lack of the 3'-OH group then
inhibits further elongation of DNA.*

*Mammalian polymerase is less likely to "mistake" AZT for
thymidine.*

4.41.) PURINES

Purines can either be made from scratch ("de novo") from amino acids, or they can be recycled. Recycling is especially important for tissues with rapid cell turnover (blood cells, epithelia…)

A) De novo synthesis (in liver):

1.) | phosphoribosyl pyrophosphate | → | IMP |

2.) | IMP | → | AMP or GMP | → | ADP or GDP |

B) Salvage of purine bases (recycling):

| hypoxanthine | → | IMP |

| guanine | → | GMP |

| adenine | → | AMP |

 Lesch-Nyhan: *Defective phosphoribosyl transferase: Purine bases cannot be salvaged and are all degraded to uric acid → gout, severe neurological signs.*

C) Degradation of purine bases (in liver):

1.) | adenosine | → | inosine | → | hypoxanthine | → | xanthine |

      | guanosine | → | guanine | → | xanthine |

2.) | xanthine | → | uric acid |

 Allopurinol *inhibits conversion of xanthine to uric acid and is used for treatment of gout.*

4.42.) PYRIMIDINES

Like the purines, pyrimidines can be made "from scratch" or recycled:

A) De novo synthesis (in liver):

1.) $\boxed{\text{glutamine}} \rightarrow \boxed{\text{carbamoylphosphate}} \rightarrow \boxed{\text{OMP}} \rightarrow \boxed{\text{UMP}}$

2.) $\boxed{\text{UTP}} \rightarrow \boxed{\text{CTP}}$

  $\boxed{\text{dUMP}} \rightarrow \text{dTMP}$

 5-Fluorouracil (anti cancer drug) is converted by these same enzymes to 5-FdUMP which is a potent inhibitor of thymidine synthesis.

B) Salvage of pyrimidine bases (recycling):

$\boxed{\text{uracil}} \rightarrow \boxed{\text{UMP}}$

$\boxed{\text{cytosine}} \rightarrow \boxed{\text{CMP}}$

C) Degradation of pyrimidine bases (in liver):

Pyrimidine ring can be opened and completely degraded:

$\boxed{\text{cytosine}} \rightarrow CO_2, NH_4^+$ and β-alanine

$\boxed{\text{thymine}} \rightarrow CO_2, NH_4^+$ and β-aminoisobutyrate

 These degradation products are harmless and excreted in the urine.

4.43.) GENE EXPRESSION

When studying molecular biology, you must pay close attention to differences between prokaryotes and eukaryotes. While the principles are the same, the details are quite different.

A) BACTERIA (PROKARYOTES):

operon (DNA)	• operational unit that is either "on" or "off" • consists of promoter, operator and one or more structural genes
promoter (DNA)	• RNA polymerase binds to promoter • located 5'-end of operon ("upstream")
operator (DNA)	• located between promoter and structural genes • binding site of repressors • if repressor binds to operator, the operon is "off" (polymerase can't proceed)
repressor (protein)	• regulatory protein that binds to operator and prevents transcription
regulator gene (DNA)	• codes for repressor

---

lac-OPERON:
➢ Metabolite (lactose) binds to repressor preventing its interaction with DNA.
➢ Operon freed of repressor is switched "on" and polymerase begins transcription of structural genes.
➢ Gene products: β-galactosidase plus two other proteins

B) HUMANS (EUKARYOTES):

- No operon. Each structural gene has its own promoter containing many different response elements (binding sites for regulatory proteins).

- Regulatory proteins can bind to several promoters activating a set of structural genes (which may be located on different chromosomes).

- Transcription is regulated by various combinations of regulatory proteins.

transcription factor	• binds to TATA box (part of promoter) • RNA polymerase does not recognize promoter in absence of transcription factor!
inducers	• example: steroid hormones • bind to nuclear receptor protein • inducer-receptor complex binds to DNA and activates some gene, inactivates others
enhancers	• regulatory DNA sequence • can be upstream or downstream of promoter • may be located several thousand base pairs from starting point of transcription • loops in DNA bring enhancers near the promoter region of the gene

4.44.) TRANSCRIPTION
DNA → RNA

mRNA are the "working copies" of the DNA. While cells from different tissues of the body have the same DNA, they differ in their gene expression and have different sets of mRNA. If you want to know which genes are active, you can make a cDNA library (complimentary DNA synthesized to all mRNA present in a cell).

A) BACTERIA (PROKARYOTES):

holoenzyme	• core enzyme plus σ-factor
σ-factors	• bind to RNA polymerase. • depending on σ-factor, RNA polymerase • recognizes certain promoters but not others
cistron	• region of DNA that encodes a single protein

 Prokaryotic mRNA is polycistronic (encodes multiple proteins).

B) HUMANS (EUKARYOTES):

polymerase I	• makes rRNA
polymerase II	• makes mRNA
polymerase III	• makes tRNA

Eukaryotic mRNA is heavily processed in the nucleus:
1. 5'-cap (methylated GTP) is added.
2. Poly (A) tail is added to 3' end.
3. Introns are removed and exons are spliced together.

4.45.) REPLICATION

DNA → DNA

Replication of eukaryotic DNA is "semiconservative": parental strands separate and each serves as a template for a newly synthesized one.

DNA polymerases cannot initiate synthesis of a new strand but require a primer (short oligonucleotide sequence composed of RNA). The primer is later replaced by DNA.

> ➤ Parental strand is read in 3' to 5' direction.
> ➤ New strand is produced in 5' to 3' direction.

A) BACTERIA (PROKARYOTES):

helicase	• separates parental DNA
primase	• RNA polymerase that copies parental strand and makes RNA primer
polymerase III	• major DNA polymerase • replicates both parental strands • has proofreading ability • has 3' exonuclease activity to remove wrong nucleotides
polymerase I	• removes primer and fills gap with DNA (5' exonuclease activity)
polymerase II	• DNA repair (3' exonuclease activity)
ligase	• joins Okazaki fragments of lagging strand

B) <u>HUMANS (EUKARYOTES):</u>

δ	<ul><li>major DNA polymerase</li><li>produces leading strand</li><li>also has helicase activity!</li></ul><ul><li>○ *no proofreading*</li><li>○ *no exonuclease activity*</li></ul>
α	<ul><li>DNA polymerase</li><li>produces lagging strand</li></ul><ul><li>○ *also has primase activity!*</li></ul>
β, ε	<ul><li>minor DNA polymerases</li><li>DNA repair (3′ exonuclease activity)</li></ul>
γ	<ul><li>mitochondrial DNA polymerase</li></ul>
ligase	<ul><li>joins Okazaki fragments of lagging strand</li></ul>

> ➤ **Endonuclease:** Incision of DNA
> ➤ **Exonuclease:** Removal of nucleotides from incised end

ANATOMY

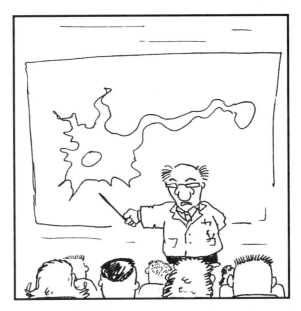

"There are 14 billion neurons in the brain and 14 billion *and one* facts to remember to pass the Boards."

Part A : Embryology

5.1.) <u>GERM LAYERS</u>

All tissues are derived from 3 embryonal germ cell layers. Adenomas and carcinomas develop in organs derived from ecto- or endoderm, sarcomas and fibromas in organs derived from the mesoderm.

ECTODERM	• **neural tube** → CNS • **neural crest** → peripheral nervous system • **placodes** → sensory organs • **surface** epithelium → skin
MESODERM	• **somites** → muscles, vertebral column • connective tissue • lymphatic tissues • blood cells
ENDODERM	• epithelium of GI tract • liver • pancreas • thymus • thyroid

5.2.) FETAL REMNANTS

The umbilical cord contains 2 arteries (deoxygenated blood) and 1 vein (oxygenated blood from placenta). The yolk stalk connects the yolk sac with the GI tract, the urachus connects the urinary bladder with the allantois. These fetal structures disappear and leave remnants.

umbilical arteries	medial umbilical ligaments
urachus	median umbilical ligament
umbilical vein	round ligament
ductus venosus	venous ligament
ductus arteriosus	ligamentum arteriosus
yolk stalk	Meckel's diverticulum

> ### Meckel's diverticulum: "2-2-2"
> - persists in **2%** of persons
> - located at antimesenteric border of ileum (within **2** feet of the ileocecal junction)
> - is about **2** cm long
>
> *Inflammation may mimic appendicitis!*

5.3.) DERIVATES OF BRANCHIAL ARCHES

Branchial arches form the pharynx-neck region (gills) of vertebrates. Each arch consists of a mesenchymal core covered by ectoderm (outside) and endoderm (inside) and gives rise to a specific bone, muscle, artery and nerve:

	BONES	MUSCLES	ARTERIES	NERVES
1st Arch mandibular arch (Meckel)	malleus incus	muscles of mastication	facial artery	V3
2nd Arch hyoid arch (Reichert)	stapes styloid lesser horns of hyoid	muscles of facial expression	ext. carotid artery	VII
3rd Arch thyrohyoid arch	body of hyoid	stylopharyngeal muscle	int. carotid artery	IX
4th Arch	larynx	pharyngeal muscles		X

PHARYNGEAL CLEFTS:

I: (between arch I and II) - forms external auditory meatus

II-IV: - cervical sinus (disappears, but may form cervical cysts)

5.4.) PHARYNGEAL POUCHES

Each of the pharyngeal clefts separating the branchial arches has a corresponding pouch on the inside. The clefts disappear (except for I), the pouches give off specialized tissues:

	TISSUES DERIVED FROM POUCHES
I	tympanic cavity eustachian tube
II	palatine tonsil
III	ventral : thymus dorsal : <u>inferior</u> parathyroids
IV	ventral : - dorsal : <u>superior</u> parathyroids
V	ultimobranchial body → parafollicular C cells of thyroid

__Cervical cysts:__
- *uncommon remnants of pharyngeal clefts*
- *located in anterolateral part of neck*
- *1-2 inches in diameter*

5.5.) <u>UROGENITAL DEVELOPMENT</u>

Up to the 7th week, the embryo is ambisexual and contains both Wolff and Müller ducts:

	MALE	FEMALE
Wolff [1]	• epididymis • vas deferens	disappears
Müller [2]	disappears	• fallopian tubes • uterus • vagina down to hymen

[1] *= mesonephric duct*
[2] *= paramesonephric duct*

<u>MALE DIFFERENTIATION:</u>
Wolff is sustained by testosterone (from Leydig cells)
Müller is suppressed by MIF glycoprotein (from Sertoli cells)

---

allantois →	• urinary bladder • urachus
ureteric bud [1] →	• bladder trigonum • ureter • collecting tubules
pronephros	(disappears, never functional)
mesonephros	(disappears, temporarily functional)
metanephros	• kidneys

[1] *inferior part of mesonephric duct (= metanephric duct)*

Part B : Gross Anatomy

5.6.) THE SKULL AND ITS HOLES

optic canal	• optic nerve • ophthalmic artery
superior orbital fissure	• cranial nerves III, IV, V (ophthalmic), VI • sympathetic nerves • ophthalmic veins
foramen rotundum	• cranial nerve V (maxillary)
foramen ovale	• cranial nerve V (mandibular) • accessory meningeal artery
foramen spinosum	• middle meningeal artery
foramen magnum	• spinal cord • accessory nerve • vertebral arteries • spinal arteries
jugular foramen	• cranial nerves IX, X, XI • internal jugular vein
hypoglossal canal	• cranial nerve XII
internal auditory meatus	• cranial nerves VII, VIII • labyrinthine artery

 Basilar skull fractures: bruises over mastoid process or periorbital.

5.7.) EYE

The eye is moved by 6 external muscles, innervated by 3 cranial nerves:

A) EXTERNAL MUSCLES:

MUSCLE	MOVES EYE:	INNERVATION
med. rectus	nasal	III (oculomotor)
lat. rectus	temporal	VI (abducens)

combined action raises eye upward:

sup. rectus	**up and nasal** rotates medially	III
inf. oblique	**up and temporal** rotates laterally	III

combined action lowers eye downward:

inf. rectus	**down and nasal** rotates laterally	III
sup. oblique	**down and temporal** rotates medially	IV (trochlear)

Abducens paralysis: *→ unable to abduct eye on affected side*
→ diplopia (double vision)

Trochlear paralysis: *→ slight vertical double image*
→ patient compensates by tilting head

B) <u>INTERNAL MUSCLES</u>:

	FUNCTION	INNERVATION
dilator pupillae	mydriasis	sympathetic
sphincter pupillae	miosis	parasympathetic
ciliary muscle	accommodation	parasympathetic

 Contraction of the ciliary muscle relaxes suspensory ligaments and allows lens to turn into globular shape for near vision.

C) <u>UPPER EYELIDS</u>:

	FUNCTION	INNERVATION
levator palpebrae sup.	raises lid	III (oculomotor)
Müller's muscle	raises lid	sympathetic

 Drowsiness → reduced sympathetic tone
→ Müller's muscles relax
→ eyelids droop

HORNER'S SYNDROME:
caused by neck injuries or tumors interrupting cervical sympathetic chain
1. *miosis* (small pupils)
2. *ptosis* (drooping eyelid)
3. red and dry facial skin on affected side

5.8.) TONGUE

A) MUSCLES:

The tongue is moved by three muscles, all of which are innervated by the hypoglossal nerve (XII):

MUSCLES	FUNCTION
genioglossus	pulls tongue out
styloglossus	pulls tongue in and up
hyoglossus	pulls tongue down

DAMAGE TO HYPOGLOSSAL NERVE (XII):
- genioglossus muscle of healthy side becomes dominant
- tongue will deviate towards side of damage

B) SENSATION:

The tongue receives sensory innervation from 3 cranial nerves:

	TASTE	TOUCH, TEMPERATURE
anterior 2/3	VII	V3
posterior 1/3	IX	IX

5.9.) <u>MANDIBLE</u>

The mandible is the largest and strongest bone in the face. In old age it atrophies somewhat as teeth are lost. The mandible and the muscles that move it are derived from the 1st branchial arch.

MUSCLES	FUNCTION
• lat. pterygoid • digastric • geniohyoid	open mouth
• masseter • medial pterygoid • temporalis	close mouth
• lateral pterygoid	protrudes mandible
• temporalis	retracts mandible
• lateral pterygoid	lateral displacement

 A blow to the jaw may fracture the neck of the mandible and/or the region of the opposite canine tooth.

5.10.) <u>LARYNX</u>

The larynx consists of 4 cartilages: The cricoid and thyroid cartilages plus a pair of arytenoid cartilages to which the vocal cords are attached. The epiglottis cartilage forms the roof and protects the larynx during swallowing.

A) <u>MUSCLES</u>:

	FUNCTION	INNERVATION
post. cricoarytenoid	opens glottis	recurrent nerve
lat. cricoarytenoid	closes glottis	recurrent nerve
thyroarytenoid	relaxes vocal chords	recurrent nerve
cricothyroid	tightens vocal chords	sup. laryngeal nerve

> ## <u>Recurrent nerves are vulnerable to injury</u>:
> - thyroidectomy
> - carotid endarterectomy
> - other operations in anterior triangle of the neck
>
> unilateral damage → hoarseness
> bilateral damage → dyspnea
>
> **Left recurrent** nerve wraps around aortic arch
> **Right recurrent** nerve wraps around right subclavian artery

B) <u>SENSATION</u>: These nerves are important to initiate the cough reflex.

above glottis	sup. laryngeal nerve
below glottis	recurrent nerve

5.11.) SHOULDER

Many muscles are involved in every movement. This chart lists only the <u>main</u> muscle responsible for each movement:

FUNCTION	MAIN MUSCLE	INNERVATION
adduction	pectoralis major	C5-T1
abduction	first 60 degrees: deltoid then: serratus anterior	long thoracic nerve
anteversion	deltoid	axillary nerve
retroversion	teres major	subscapular nerve
outward rotation	infraspinatus	suprascapular nerve
inward rotation	subscapular	subscapular nerve

"SCAPULAR WINGING" (paralysis of anterior serratus muscle):
- damage to the long thoracic nerve (stab wounds, thoracic surgery)
- medial border of scapula stands out when the person presses his arm anteriorly against a wall.

ROTATOR CUFF: supraspinatus infraspinatus
teres minor subscapularis

- These muscles hold the head of humerus in glenoid cavity of scapula.
- Injury results in instability of shoulder joint.

Inflammation of subacromial bursa → pain intensifies by abduction.

5.12.) <u>BRACHIAL PLEXUS</u>

You don't need to know every detail about the brachial plexus. There are 3 trunks distributing to 5 major nerves:

SPINAL RAMI	TRUNKS	TERMINAL NERVES
C5 - C6	upper trunk	musculocutaneous nerve
C7	middle trunk	axillary nerve radial nerve median nerve
C8 - T1	lower trunk	ulnar nerve

┌┄┄┄┄┄┐
└┄┄┄┄┄┘ = posterior cord

5.13.) <u>BRACHIAL PLEXUS INJURIES</u>

These occur sometimes during delivery of a baby, if you pull the arm too much...

upper brachial plexus injury	• forceful separation of neck and shoulder • motorcycle accidents, football tackling • arm hangs in medial rotation **("waiter's tip position")**
posterior cord injury	• compression by too long crutches • radial nerve injury **("wrist drop")**
lower brachial plexus injury	• forceful pull of arm/shoulders (birth) • ulnar nerve injury **("claw hand")**

5.14.) BRACHIAL NERVE INJURIES

Injury to brachial nerves results in characteristic motor and sensory deficits:

	NERVE INJURY RESULTS IN:
radial nerve	• **"wrist drop"** • loss of triceps reflex o *sensory loss: posterior arm, dorsal hand*
median nerve	• no flexion of thumb, index and middle finger • no thumb opposition • thenar atrophy o *sensory loss: radial 2½ fingers (palm and tips)*
ulnar nerve	• **"claw hand"** • no flexion of 4th and 5th finger • apothenar atrophy o *sensory loss: ulnar 1½ fingers (palm and tips)*
musculocutaneous n.	• no elbow flexion • no supination • loss of biceps reflex o *sensory loss: extensor aspect of forearm*

Carpal tunnel syndrome: Compression of <u>median nerve</u> by carpal ligament.
→ pain/tingling in distribution area of median nerve
(often most bothersome at night)

Humerus fracture: Risk of <u>radial nerve</u> injury (spirals down near humerus).

5.15.) <u>ELBOW</u>

This chart lists only the <u>main</u> muscle responsible for each movement:

FUNCTION	MAIN MUSCLE	INNERVATION
flexion	biceps brachii	musculocutaneous nerve
extension	triceps brachii	radial nerve
supination [1]	biceps brachii	musculocutaneous nerve
pronation [2]	pronator teres	median nerve

[1] *palm faces anteriorly, thumb points to lateral side*
[2] *palm faces posteriorly, thumb points to medial side*

"Tennis elbow":
- repetitive stress, especially "backhand play"
- due to inflammation of the lateral epicondyle, which is the origin of extensor muscles of the forearm.
- the elbow joint and olecranon are NOT involved!

Colles' fracture: *Fracture of radius near wrist*
→ *dorsal/lateral position of hand*

5.16.) <u>HIP</u>

This chart lists only the <u>main</u> muscle responsible for each movement:

FUNCTION	MAIN MUSCLE	INNERVATION
outward rotation	gluteus maximus	inf. gluteal nerve
inward rotation	gluteus medius / minimus	sup. gluteal nerve
extension	gluteus maximus	inf. gluteal nerve
flexion	iliopsoas	femoral nerve
abduction	gluteus medius	sup. gluteal nerve
adduction	adductor magnus / minimus	obturator nerve

Pelvic fractures:	• automobile accidents • risk of severe internal bleeding
Femur neck fractures:	• common in elderly women (osteoporosis) • risk of femur head necrosis • significant morbidity / mortality

Femur neck fracture: *the leg is abducted and externally rotated.*

5.17.) <u>KNEE</u>

This chart lists only the <u>main</u> muscle responsible for each movement:

FUNCTION	MAIN MUSCLE	INNERVATION
extension	quadriceps femoris	femoral nerve
flexion	"<u>hamstrings</u>": • semimembranous muscle • semitendinous muscle • biceps femoris	sciatic nerve
inward rotation	semimembranous	sciatic nerve
outward rotation	biceps femoris	sciatic nerve

<u>PULLED HAMSTRINGS:</u>
- Common sports injury in persons who run and kick balls
- Tearing of fibers → very painful

<u>KNEE INJURY:</u>
- Rupture of anterior cruciate ligament: tibia can be drawn anteriorly.
- Rupture of posterior cruciate ligament: tibia can be drawn posteriorly.
- Rupture of lateral ligaments: tibia can be bend laterally.
- Meniscus injuries: pain upon extension of flexed knee (McMurray's test).

The gluteal region is a common side for IM injection of drugs.
- risk of sciatic nerve injury
- upper lateral quadrant is safer

5.18.) ANKLE

Notice how each muscle moves the ankle in 2 axes. Movement in one axis alone requires combined action of two muscles:

MUSCLE	FUNCTION	INNERVATION
tibialis anterior	dorsiflexes + *inverts foot*	deep peroneal nerve
peroneus tertius	dorsiflexes + *everts foot*	deep peroneal nerve
peroneus longus and brevis	plantarflexes + *inverts foot*	superficial peroneal n.
tibialis posterior	plantarflexes + *everts foot*	tibial nerve

INJURY TO COMMON PERONEAL NERVE:
- winds around neck of fibula
- most commonly injured nerve of lower limb
- loss of dorsiflexion → "foot drop"

INJURY TO TIBIAL NERVE:
- rare (deep laceration of popliteal fossa)
- inability to plantarflex foot and toes

FRACTURES OF TIBIA:
- "bumper fractures"
- skin tears → frequent compound fractures

5.19.) MEDIASTINUM

The mediastinum is the space between the lungs (lateral), the sternum (anterior) and the vertebral column (posterior).

A) SUPERIOR MEDIASTINUM:

	CONTENT
superior mediastinum	• thymus • great vessels of heart • trachea • esophagus

B) INFERIOR MEDIASTINUM:

middle mediastinum	• heart
posterior (of heart) mediastinum	• esophagus • descending aorta
anterior (of heart) mediastinum	• large during infancy (filled by thymus) [1]

[1] in infancy is wider than the heart silhouette on X-ray!

5.20.) CORONARY ARTERIES

The heart muscle receives its blood flow from two coronary arteries that originate from the ascending aorta just above the aortic valve.

	SUPPLIES:
left coronary artery → ant. interventricular and circumflex artery	• most of the left atrium • most of the left ventricle • anterior portion of septum
right coronary artery	• right atrium • right ventricle • variable amount of left atrium and ventricle • sinus node • AV node

 Blood flow *through coronary arteries is highest during early diastole and lowest during systole!*

right dominant (85%): posterior septum supplied by right c.a.
left dominant (10%): posterior septum supplied by left c.a.
mixed (5%)

5.21.) ABDOMINAL ARTERIES

Arterial infarctions are rare because these vessels have many anastomoses. Infarction of the bowels is usually due to interruption of venous drainage.

	BRANCHES	ORGANS
celiac trunk	• left gastric artery • splenic artery • hepatic artery • gastroduodenal artery • sup. pancreaticoduodenal art.	• stomach • spleen • liver • proximal duodenum
sup. mesenteric art.	inf. pancreaticoduodenal art. many branches	• distal duodenum • small intestine • cecum • ascending colon • transverse colon
inf. mesenteric art.	many branches superior rectal artery	• descending colon • sigmoid • rectum

PORTOCAVAL SHUNTS:

gastric/esophageal veins →	esophageal varices
anorectal veins →	hemorrhoids
paraumbilical veins →	caput medusae

5.22.) <u>PERITONEUM</u>

The peritoneum is a serous membrane that covers the entire wall and wraps over the viscera contained in it. In men, it forms a closed sac. In women it is pierced by the uterine tubes.

INTRAPERITONEAL	RETROPERITONEAL
• stomach • small bowel • transverse colon • spleen o part of liver	• aorta • vena cava • kidneys • pancreas • duodenum • ascending colon • descending colon

<u>ACUTE APPENDICITIS</u>:

McBurney's point: at junction between lateral and middle thirds of a line between umbilicus and anterior superior iliac spine.

<u>Signs of peritonitis:</u>
severe pain (localized or diffuse)
rebound tenderness
abdominal muscle rigidity

5.23.) LAYERS OF SPERMATIC CORD

Since the inguinal canal is formed by the descending testis, it is easy to see how the layers of the spermatic cord are derived from the layers of the abdominal wall:

deep	
loose connective tissue	arteries, pampiniform plexus
internal spermatic fascia	from fascia transversalis
cremaster muscle and fascia	from int. oblique muscle
external spermatic fascia	from ext. oblique aponeurosis
superficial fascia	contains dartos muscle
superficial	

5.24.) OVARY / TESTIS

"Important organs receive multiple blood supplies.":

ovary	• aorta → ovarian artery • internal iliac a. → uterine artery
testis	• aorta → testicular artery • internal iliac a. → art. of ductus deferens • inf. epigastric a. → cremasteric artery

250

Part C : Neuroanatomy

5.25.) CORTEX

The two hemispheres are connected by the corpus callosum. Patients with complete transection of the corpus have subtle cognitive deficits relating verbal expression of non-verbal input:

LEFT HEMISPHERE	RIGHT HEMISPHERE
• language • mathematics • sequential • analytical	• non-verbal • musical • geometrical • spatial comprehension

vision	occipital lobe
hearing	temporal lobe
taste	insula, below postcentral gyrus
reading, writing	angular gyrus
primary motor cortex	precentral gyrus
primary sensory cortex	postcentral gyrus
Wernicke (sensory)	temporal lobe, superior gyrus
Broca (motor)	frontal lobe, near lateral fissure

APHASIAS:
Broca: nonfluent speech, good comprehension
Wernicke: fluent but nonsensical speech, poor comprehension

5.26.) CEREBRAL ARTERIES

Stroke: 80% ischemic, 20% hemorrhagic

The circle of Willis receives blood supply from the 2 carotid arteries and the basilar artery. It gives rise to 3 pairs of cerebral arteries:

	SUPPLIES:	OCCLUSION RESULTS IN:
ant. cerebral a.	medial cortex	motor & sensory loss *(contralateral legs and feet)*
middle cerebral a.	lateral cortex ant. limb of internal capsule	motor & sensory loss *(contralateral upper body)*
post. cerebral a.	occipital cortex	homonymous hemianopsia *(contralateral)*
ant. choroidal a.	basal ganglia hypothalamus post. limb of internal capsule	
cerebellar aa.	cerebellum lateral portions of brain stem	ataxia brainstem syndromes

homonymous hemianopsia:

left   right

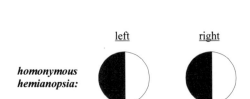

5.27.) TRANSIENT ISCHEMIC ATTACKS

TIAs are caused by partial occlusion of cerebral arteries by plaques or emboli. They may be precursors to a full stroke and it is important to recognize the symptoms:

INTERNAL CAROTID ARTERY	VERTEBROBASILAR ARTERY
o ipsilateral monocular blindness ("amaurosis fugax") o hemiparesis, contralateral o hemisensory loss, contralateral o language disturbance	o vertigo o diplopia o ataxia o facial numbness/weakness o nausea

5.28.) HYPERTENSIVE HEMORRHAGE

HEMORRHAGE INTO:	RESULTS IN:
putamen	• contralateral weakness, including face • contralateral hemianopsia
thalamus	• contralateral hemiparesis • sensory changes • homonymous hemianopsia
pons	• coma • small reactive pupils • quadriplegia
cerebellum	• unsteady gait • clumsiness • nausea, vomiting

5.29.) CRANIAL NERVES

Most cranial nerves carry both motor and sensory functions. Visceral motor nerves form the "autonomic nervous system".

A) MOTOR:

	NERVE	FUNCTIONS
somatic motor	III	• extraocular eye muscles (except sup. oblique and lat. rectus)
	IV	• superior oblique
	VI	• lateral rectus
	XII	• tongue muscles (except palatoglossus)
branchial motor (derived from branchial arches)	V	• mastication
	VII	• facial expression
	IX, X	• pharynx, larynx
	XI	• trapezius, sternocleidomastoid muscles
visceral motor	III	• ciliary muscle, constrictor pupillae
	VII	• all glands except parotid
	IX	• parotid
	X	• abdominal viscera up to splenic flexure

B) SENSORY:

	NERVE	FUNCTIONS
special sensory	I	• smell
	II	• vision
	VII, IX	• taste
	VIII	• hearing, balance
general sensory	V, VII, IX, X	• pain, temperature, touch, proprioception
visceral sensory	IX, X	• afferents for visceral reflexes

5.30.) PARASYMPATHETIC GANGLIA

The parasympathetic nervous system has a cranial and a sacral component. No parasympathetic fibers originate in the cervical, thoracic or lumbar segments. This chart summarizes the functions of the cranial portion of the parasympathetic nervous system:

NUCLEUS	NERVE	GANGLION	ORGANS
Edinger-Westphal	III	ciliary	eye
sup. salivary nucleus	VII	sublingual submaxillary	lacrimal gland nasal glands submandibular gland
inf. salivary nucleus	IX	otic	parotid gland
dorsal motor nucleus	X	many, mostly intramural	many

Pupillary light reflex: *Optical nerve → tectal area → Edinger-Westphal nucleus → parasympathetic → sphincter*
Argyll-Robertson pupil: *Damage to tectal area (e.g. syphilis): pupils constrict for near vision but not for light.*

5.31.) BASAL GANGLIA

The basal ganglia receive input from all parts of the cortex and project via thalamus to the precentral motor cortex. They are involved in the programming of movement.

striatum	• caudate • putamen • globus pallidus
neostriatum	• caudate • putamen
paleostriatum	• globus pallidus
lentiform nucleus	• putamen • globus pallidus

PARKINSON'S DISEASE:
- loss of dopaminergic input from substantia nigra to striatum
- o bradykinesia (difficulty initiating or stopping a movement)
- o muscle rigidity
- o tremor ("pill-rolling")

HUNTINGTON'S DISEASE:
- atrophy of caudate nucleus
- o chorea: involuntary movements
- o personality changes, dementia

WILSON'S DISEASE:
- copper accumulation in lentiform nucleus (and elsewhere)
- o tremor, spasticity, chorea, bizarre behavior

5.32.) <u>THALAMUS</u>

> "Thalamus knows all" (receives all sensory input, except olfactory)

The thalamus is the major sensory relay station of the brain. Thalamic-cortical interactions determine consciousness and the sleep/wake cycle.

I.) ANTERIOR THALAMUS (part of limbic system)	input: mammillary bodies output: cingula (cortex)
II.) LATERAL THALAMUS	major nucleus: "pulvinar"
ventral anterior nucleus	receives input from basal ganglia output to premotor cortex
ventral posterior nucleus	**VPL:** medial lemniscus, spinothalamic tract (proprioception, touch) **VPM:** trigeminal nerve (taste)
ventrolateral nucleus	input from cerebellum and basal ganglia output to motor cortex
III.) MEDIAL THALAMUS	projects to frontal cortex
IV.) POSTERIOR THALAMUS	**medial geniculate:** auditory pathway **lateral geniculate:** optic tract

> <u>General features of thalamus:</u>
> - major synaptic relay station (sensory input)
> - basal ganglia → thalamus → cortex
> - rhythm established by thalamus forms major contribution to EEG

Some patients with thalamic injury become insensitive to pain and other sensory stimuli.

5.33.) BRAINSTEM SYNDROMES

Brainstem syndromes are complex because many structures are packed tightly together in a small space. The most famous one is the <u>Wallenberg syndrome</u> (lateral medulla infarction due to occlusion of posterior inferior cerebellar artery).

	BLOOD SUPPLY
medulla	lateral: posterior inferior cerebellar artery medial: anterior spinal artery
lower pons	lateral: anterior inferior cerebellar artery medial: basilar artery
upper pons	lateral: superior cerebellar artery medial: basilar artery

 The brainstem contains vital centers (respiratory and cardiovascular) and the reticular activating system that projects to the thalamus and determines consciousness. A crude way to assess brainstem function in your patients is to check their pupillary light reflex.

5.34.) MEDULLA

| Infarction of lateral medulla: | = Wallenberg |

DAMAGE TO:	RESULTS IN:
spinal tract nucleus V	ipsilateral face: pain / temp loss
nucleus solitarius	ipsilateral tongue: loss of taste
reticular formation	ipsilateral Horner's syndrome
nucleus ambiguus	hoarseness loss of pharyngeal reflex
spinothalamic tract	contralateral body pain / temp loss

Infarction of medial medulla:

DAMAGE TO:	RESULTS IN:
hypoglossal muscle	ipsilateral tongue: atrophic paralysis
medial lemniscus	contralateral loss of position sense contralateral loss of vibration sense
pyramidal tract	contralateral body: spastic paralysis

5.35.) LOWER PONS

Infarction of lateral pons:

DAMAGE TO:	RESULTS IN:
spinocerebellar tract	ipsilateral limb ataxia
nucleus VII	ipsilateral face: paralysis
spinal tract nucleus V	ipsilateral face: loss of sensation
reticular formation	ipsilateral Horner's syndrome
vestibular nucleus	vertigo
cochlear nuclei	deafness / tinnitus

Infarction of medial pons:

DAMAGE TO:	RESULTS IN:
nucleus VII	ipsilateral face: spastic paralysis
medial long. fasciculus	ipsilateral eye can not adduct on lateral gaze
nucleus VI	ipsilateral paralysis of lat. rectus oculi
corticospinal tract	contralateral body: spastic paralysis
medial lemniscus	contralateral loss of position and vibration sense

5.36.) UPPER PONS

Infarction of lateral pons:

DAMAGE TO:	RESULTS IN:
motor nucleus V	ipsilateral loss of masseter function
reticular formation	ipsilateral Horner's syndrome
spinothalamic tract	contralateral loss of pain and sensation

Infarction of medial pons:

DAMAGE TO:	RESULTS IN:
corticospinal tract	contralateral spastic paralysis

5.37.) WHERE IS THE LESION?

A large part of neurology is to localize the lesion based on your knowledge of neuroanatomy.

TYPICAL SYMPTOMS	LESION
Loss of pain and temperature sensation arms and shoulder	Syringomyelia
Muscle weakness and loss of sensation in left arm	Right middle cerebral a.
Muscle weakness and loss of sensation in left leg	Right anterior cerebral a.
Spastic paralysis, loss of proprioception left leg and loss of pain and temperature sensation right leg	Hemisection of left spinal cord
Spastic paralysis both legs	Total transection of spinal cord
Flaccid paralysis, loss of sensations, both legs	Guillain-Barré syndrome
Muscle atrophy, fasciculations both arms & legs	ALS
Loss of pain and temperature sensation left arms, legs, body Paralysis of left arms, legs and body Loss of sensation right lower face	"Wallenberg syndrome" (right lateral medulla)
Sensory loss both hands and feet ("sock&glove pattern")	Peripheral neuropathy
Loss of sensation over buttocks, perineum and impotence	Cauda equina lesion

5.38.) KEY DERMATOMES

skull	C2
thumb	C6
nipple	T5
belly button	T10
big toe	L4
penis	S3
anus	S5
knee jerk reflex	L4
ankle jerk reflex	S1

 The lowest segment (S5) is around the anus, not the toes!

263

PHYSIOLOGY

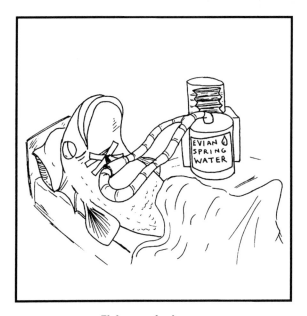

Fish respirators.

6.1.) SIX EQUATIONS YOU REALLY NEED

1. HOW TO CALCULATE TOTAL PERIPHERAL RESISTANCE:

Mean blood pressure $\quad P_{average} = P_{diastolic} + 1/3\ (P_{systolic} - P_{diastolic})$

Total peripheral resistance $\quad$ TPR = mean blood pressure / cardiac output

EXAMPLE: $\qquad$ systolic blood pressure 120 mmHg
$\qquad$ diastolic blood pressure 80 mmHg
$\qquad$ cardiac output 5,000 mL/min

$\qquad \rightarrow$ mean pressure = 80 + 1/3 (120-80) = 93 mmHg
$\qquad \rightarrow$ TPR = 93/5,000 = 0.018

Norepinephrine increases TPR (α-receptors $\rightarrow$ vasoconstriction)
Epinephrine decreases TPR (β-receptors $\rightarrow$ vasodilation)

2. HOW TO CALCULATE CARDIAC OUTPUT:

Cardiac output = systemic blood flow = pulmonary blood flow
(Assuming that there are no intracardiac shunts!)

Fick's Principle: $\quad$ pulmonary flow = oxygen uptake / (a-v oxygen difference)

EXAMPLE: $\qquad$ arterial O_2 = 20 mL oxygen / 100 mL blood = 0.2
$\qquad$ venous O_2 = 15 mL oxygen / 100 mL blood = 0.15
$\qquad$ oxygen uptake = 250 mL / min

$\qquad \rightarrow$ cardiac output = 250 / 0.05 = 5,000 mL / min

Cardiac output is usually normalized to body surface area (= "cardiac index").

3. HOW TO CALCULATE RENAL CLEARANCE:

Clearance of X   clearance $\cdot$ [X]$_{plasma}$ = urine flow $\cdot$ [X]$_{urine}$

EXAMPLE: plasma creatinine concentration = 1.5 mg/dL
urine creatinine concentration = 180 mg/dL
urine flow = 1,500 mL / 24 h $\approx$ 1 mL/min

$\rightarrow$ creatinine clearance = 1 mL/min (180/1.5) = 120 mL/min

4. ACID / BASE CALCULATIONS:

Henderson-Hasselbalch $pH = pK + \log \dfrac{[salt]}{[acid]}$

$pH = 6.1 + \log \dfrac{[HCO_3^-]}{[CO_2]}$

$pH = 6.1 + \log \dfrac{[HCO_3^-]}{0.03 \, PCO_2}$

EXAMPLE: plasma bicarbonate = 24 mM/L
PCO$_2$ = 40 mmHg

$\rightarrow$ pH = 6.1 + log (24/1.2) = 6.1 + log (20) = 7.4

Bicarbonate is a powerful buffer (despite having a pK 6.1 far from physiological pH) because the acid ($H_2CO_3 \leftrightarrow CO_2$) and salt ($HCO_3^-$) concentrations are independently regulated by the body:
- *Kidneys regulate HCO_3^-*
- *Lung ventilation regulates CO_2*

---

log 0.1 = -1   /   log 1 = 0   /   log 10 = 1   /   log 100 = 2 etc....

---

5. HOW TO CALCULATE DIFFUSION CAPACITY OF THE LUNG:

Diffusion (Fick's law) $\text{flow} = D \cdot \text{area} \cdot \dfrac{\text{concentration gradient}}{\text{membrane thickness}}$

Since lung area and membrane thickness of the lung cannot be measured directly, they are lumped together with the diffusion coefficient:

$$\text{flow} = D_L \cdot \text{concentration gradient}$$

EXAMPLE: alveolar partial pressure of CO = 200 mmHg
blood partial pressure of CO = 0 mmHg
flow = 4,000 mL/min

→ CO diffusion capacity $D_{L_{CO}}$ = 20 mL / min · mmHg

CO_2 and O_2 equilibrate within $1/3^{rd}$ of capillary transient time (<u>perfusion limited!</u>)

CO on the other hand is less lipid soluble (<u>diffusion limited</u>) and therefore well suited for measuring diffusion properties of the lung. This is done with a single inspiration of diluted CO and measuring the rate of disappearance of CO from alveolar gas.

Increased DL: Recruitment and dilation of pulmonary capillaries.
(may double during exercise!)

Decreased DL: Interstitial lung diseases, emphysema and V/Q imbalance.

6. HOW TO CALCULATE LUNG COMPLIANCE:

Elasticity $\text{elasticity} = \dfrac{\Delta \text{ pressure}}{\Delta \text{ volume}}$

Compliance (="stretchability") $\text{compliance} = 1/\text{elasticity} = \dfrac{\Delta \text{ volume}}{\Delta \text{ pressure}}$

Patient's with COPD have lungs with <u>high</u> compliance.
Patient's with restrictive lung disease have <u>low</u> compliance.
A rod of steal has higher elasticity (less stretchability) than a rubber band.

6.2.) ION CHANNELS

Ion channels are most crucial for excitatory cells. Opening of these channels results in membrane potential moving towards the equilibrium potential for [X]. You can calculate the equilibrium potential of [X] from intracellular and extracellular [X] concentrations (Nernst).

	KEY FEATURES
K^+ channels	• maintain resting membrane potential • repolarization phase of action potentials • afterhyperpolarization
Na^+ channels	• upstroke phase of neuronal action potential • phase 0 of cardiac action potential (myocyte) • rapid inactivation → repolarization (refractory period)
Ca^{2+} channels	• excitation contraction coupling • excitation secretion coupling • phase 0 of cardiac pacemaker cells (sinus node) • cardiac plateau phase: Ca^{2+} entry • intracellular Ca^{2+} release (ryanodine receptor)
cation channels	• depolarization • dark current of photoreceptors • nicotinic ACh receptor at motor endplate
Cl^- channels	• CNS: inhibitory postsynaptic potentials
Na^+ / K^+ pump	• maintains ion gradients • is electrogenic: 3 Na^+ out for 2 K^+ in (but direct contribution to RMP is very small)

Absolute refractory period:
Action potentials cannot be generated because of inactivation of the Na^+ channels.
Relative refractory period:
Some Na^+ channels have recovered from inactivation. Strong stimuli may generate action potentials with slow upstroke and low amplitude.

6.3.) <u>TRANSPORT</u>

Lipid bilayers are permeable for water and small, uncharged molecules. Other molecules require membrane transport proteins, either carriers which take advantage of concentration gradients or pumps which derive their energy from ATP.

		TRANSPORTERS	
	PASSIVE (diffusion)	FACILITATED (carriers)	ACTIVE (pumps)
ATP required?	no	no	yes
can it transport against gradient?	no	no (yes if coupled)	yes
substrate specific?	no	yes	yes
saturating?	no	yes	yes

<u>EXAMPLES:</u>

- **Active transport:** Na^+ / K^+ ATPase
  H^+ / K^+ ATPase

- **Facilitated transport:**   simple glucose carriers

  Secondary active transport: $Na^+ /$ glucose carriers
  $Na^+ /$ amino acid carriers
  (Glucose and amino acids are transported <u>against</u> their gradients, but this is driven by Na^+ moving down its own gradient.)

- **Passive transport:**   water, electrolytes, O_2 etc.

6.4.) <u>SIGNAL TRANSDUCTION</u>

2nd messengers are generated intracellularly and amplify the signal:
- receptor → G protein → adenylyl cyclase → cAMP → protein kinase A
- nitric oxide → guanylyl cyclase → cGMP → protein kinase G
- receptor → G protein → phospholipase C → IP3. DAG → protein kinase C

	HORMONES / RECEPTORS
cAMP ↑	• β, H2 receptors • ACTH
cAMP ↓	• α2 receptors • M2, M3 receptors
cGMP ↑	• nitric oxide • ANP • Viagra^{TM} [1]
IP3, DAG	• α1, M1, M4, H1 receptors • angiotensin receptors • tachykinins • endothelin
tyrosine kinase	• insulin • growth factors
gene expression	• steroid hormones • thyroid hormones • retinoic acid

[1] inhibits type V cGMP phosphodiesterase → enhanced effect of nitric oxide on penile artery dilation.

Tyrosine kinase phosphorylates many proteins. It also activates the ras → raf → MAP kinase cascade which modulates gene expression. Out of control activation of ras is a/w with many neoplasms.

- Hormone receptor interaction first sets the timer (GDP on α-subunit is replaced by GTP), then starts it (α-subunit dissociates from β/γ).
- Activated α-subunit interacts with other enzymes such as adenylyl cyclase.
- α-subunit has built-in enzymatic activity that hydrolyzes its GTP to GDP, which terminates the action of the α-subunit ("time is up").

Gi	inhibits adenylate cyclase
Gs	stimulates adenylate cyclase
Gq	activates phospholipase C

6.5.) NERVE FIBERS

large diameter
high velocity

Aα	• efferent: skeletal muscle • afferent: from muscle spindle
Aγ	• efferent: to muscle spindle
Aβ , Aδ	• afferent: touch fast sharp pain
C	• afferent: slow dull pain
B , C	• efferent: autonomic nerves

small diameter
low velocity

"All-or-None" response:
If the stimulus is not strong enough to depolarize the membrane to threshold, no action potential occurs. If threshold is reached, a uniform action potential is generated. Stimulus strength determines frequency but not amplitude of action potentials.

6.6.) <u>TOUCH RECEPTORS</u>

Specialized receptors mediate the five sensory modalities:

A) <u>SENSORY FIBERS TRAVELLING IN DORSAL COLUMNS OF SPINAL CORD</u>:

1. pressure	• Merkel's disks *(slowly adapting)*	
2. touch	• Meissner's corpuscle *(fast adapting)* • hair follicle sensors	
3. vibration	• Pacinian corpuscle *(most rapidly adapting)*	

B) <u>SENSORY FIBERS TRAVELLING IN SPINOTHALAMIC TRACT</u>:

4. pain	• mostly free nerve endings
5. temperature	• mostly free nerve endings

***Paradoxical cold:** At temperatures > 45°C (120F) cold fibers begin to fire again (together with pain fibers). This sensation of pain and coolness is called "paradoxical cold".*

6.7.) <u>ACCOMMODATION</u>

Accommodation adjusts the lens to the distance of the object, to obtain an in-focus image on the retina. In addition, the pupils constrict when focusing a near object ("accommodation reflex").

NEAR OBJECT	FAR OBJECT
ciliary muscle contracted	ciliary muscle relaxed
zonula fibers relaxed	zonula fibers tense
lens rounded (if elastic)	lens flat
focal length short	focal length far

myopia (nearsightedness)	• lens has normal elasticity • focal point too short (or eye ball too long) *corrected with negative lens (concave)*
hypermetropia (farsightedness)	• lens has normal elasticity • focal point too far (or eye ball too short) *corrected with positive lens (convex)*
presbyopia (age)	• lens has lost elasticity • cannot shorten focal length *corrected with positive lens (convex)*

 Patients with hypermetropia and presbyopia have difficulty reading.

6.8.) NYSTAGMUS

Involuntary rhythmic movements of eyes, usually horizontal, that have a slow phase followed by a rapid snap back. Direction of nystagmus is defined by the <u>fast</u> phase.

optokinetic	• looking out of train *nystagmus against movement of image*
vestibular	• postrotational nystagmus *nystagmus against direction of prior rotation* • caloric nystagmus *nystagmus away from cold ear*
pathologic	**horizontal:** vestibular disease **vertical:** brainstem disease

 Caloric testing is used to diagnose labyrinthine disease (vertigo).

6.9.) COCHLEA

The endocochlear potential is +80 mV, as a result, hair cells have a membrane potential of −150 mV relative to scala media, making them very sensitive to permeability changes.

scala vestibuli	Na$^+$ rich	perilymph
scala media	K$^+$ rich	endolymph
scala tympani	Na$^+$ rich	perilymph

> **pitch:** frequency range 20-20,000 Hz
> **loudness:** pressure range 0-140 dB
>
> 10 dB = 10 fold change in sound intensity
> 20 dB = 100 fold change in sound intensity

6.10.) DEAFNESS

In patients with diminished hearing it is important to distinguish between middle ear versus inner ear problems. This can be done with a simple tuning fork test:

TUNING FORK TESTS:

	WEBER	RINNE
method	Place fork on top of skull	Place fork on mastoid process until tone disappears (= bone conduction). Then hold next to ear (= air conduction).
normal	Sound is equal in both ears.	Air conduction is better than bone conduction.
conduction deafness [1] (middle ear)	Sound lateralized to sick ear.	Bone conduction is better than air conduction.
nerve deafness [2] (inner ear)	Sound lateralized to normal ear.	Air conduction is better than bone conduction.

[1] chronic otitis, otosclerosis or occlusion of external auditory meatus
[2] cochlear disease or injury to cranial nerve VIII.

 Unilateral cortical lesions do NOT affect hearing since cochlear nuclei project to both temporal lobes.

6.11.) AUTONOMIC NERVOUS SYSTEM

The ANS has 3 major divisions (1.) enteric, (2.) sympathetic and (3.) parasympathetic. The sympathetic nervous system mediates the "flight or fright" response, while the parasympathetic nervous system has more discrete functions: digestion, micturition, erections, pupillary light reflex...

	SYMPATHETIC	PARASYMPATHETIC
heart	• increased heart rate • increased conduction • increased contraction	• decreased heart rate
bronchi	• dilates	• constricts
GI tract	• reduces motility	• increases motility
sphincters of GI tract	• constricts	• relaxes
rectum	• allows filling	• empties • relaxes internal sphincter
bladder	• allows filling	• empties • relaxes internal sphincter
erection		• erection
ejaculation	• triggers ejaculation	
pupils of eye	• big (mydriasis)	• small (miosis)
sweat glands	• sweat (cholinergic!)	
salivary glands		• secretion
blood vessels	• depends on receptors: - α constricts - β dilates	• dilates artery of penis only

> **Four ways to decrease blood pressure:**
> 1. block nicotinic ganglionic receptors
> 2. block β receptors
> 3. block α1 receptors
> 4. stimulate α2 receptors

6.12.) <u>CHOLINERGIC RECEPTORS</u>

There are 2 classes of cholinergic receptors (1.) nicotinic receptors stimulated by nicotine and (2.) muscarinic receptors stimulated by muscarine.

	LOCATION
nicotinic	• autonomic ganglia • sympathetic and parasympathetic ganglia! • adrenal medulla • neuromuscular junction these receptors differ from autonomic ones! SIGNAL TRANSDUCTION ligand-gated non-selective cation channel
muscarinic	• postsynaptic parasympathetic • sweat glands (innervated by sympathetic nerves!) SIGNAL TRANSDUCTION *second messenger depends on receptor subtype:* M1, M3 → PLC → IP3, DAG M2, M4 → inhibit adenylate cyclase → cAMP↓

Antagonists: Nicotinic (ganglionic):   hexamethonium
Nicotinic (motor endplate):   tubocurarine
Muscarinic: atropine

6.13.) ADRENERGIC RECEPTORS

There are 2 classes of adrenergic receptors (1.) α-receptors, which are excitatory except in the GI tract and (2.) β-receptors, which are inhibitory except at the heart.

alpha 1	• postsynaptic sympathetic • generally excitatory (vasoconstriction) • in GI tract inhibitory *Gq → phospholipase C → IP3, DAG*
alpha 2	• presynaptic sympathetic (decrease catecholamine release) • central nervous system (decrease sympathetic tone) *Gi → inhibits adenylate cyclase → cAMP↓*
beta 1	• postsynaptic sympathetic (cardiac) excitatory (chronotrope, dromotrope, inotrope) *Gs → adenylate cyclase → cAMP↑*
beta 2	• postsynaptic sympathetic (all others) inhibitory (vasodilation, bronchodilation) *Gs → adenylate cyclase → cAMP↑*

Agonists: *alpha: epinephrine ≥ norepinephrine >> isoproterenol*
        ***beta 1 :** isoproterenol > epinephrine = norepinephrine*
        ***beta 2 :** isoproterenol > epinephrine >> norepinephrine*

Vascular tone:
Norepinephrine injection → stimulates α-receptors → vasoconstriction → increase in diastolic blood pressure.

Epinephrine injection → stimulates α and β-receptors, but β-effect predominates → vasodilation → decrease in diastolic blood pressure.

6.14.) CONTROL OF HEART BEAT

The heart receives tonic input from both sympathetic and parasympathetic nerves and the heart rate depends on the balance of the two. In humans, parasympathetic tone is stronger → removal of both sympathetic. and parasympathetic innervation results in increased heart rate!

right vagus nerve	• slows frequency (sinus node)
left vagus nerve	• slows conduction (AV node) • decreased force of contraction (atria but not ventricles!)
sympathetic	• increased frequency • increased conduction • increased force of contraction (atria and ventricles)
epinephrine injection	• increased conduction and contraction • increased frequency • *increased systolic pressure* • *decreased diastolic pressure (vasodilation)*
norepinephrine injection	• increased conduction and contraction • decreased frequency (baroreceptor reflex !) • *increased systolic pressure* • *increased diastolic pressure (vasoconstriction)*

> **Frank-Starling mechanism:**
> Preload = end-diastolic volume in ventricle
> Preload↑ → muscle filament overlap↑ → stroke volume↑

6.15.) CONTROL OF MUSCLE TONE

Muscle tone is "fine-tuned" by two sensory organs:

	FUNCTION	NERVE FIBER
muscle spindle	• measures muscle length • activates α motoneuron when stretched	γ efferent 1A afferent
Golgi tendon organ	• measures muscle tension • inhibits α motoneuron	1B afferent

STRETCH REFLEX (example: knee jerk reflex): Intrafusal fibers (muscle spindle) run parallel with skeletal muscle fibers. Stretching results in firing of 1A afferent that excites the α-motoneuron (monosynaptic reflex). The α-motoneuron of the antagonistic muscle is inhibited via an interneuron.

Increased muscle tone:
- activation of γ-fibers
- upper motor neuron lesions (hemiplegia)
- Parkinson
- cold, anxiety

Decreased muscle tone:
- lower motor neuron lesions
- spinal shock (early phase of hemiplegia)
- warmth

Decorticate posture:
- legs extended, arms flexed (cortex injury)

Decerebrate posture:
- legs and arms extended (brainstem injury)

6.16.) MUSCLE TYPES

"Fast" muscles are for rapid, powerful actions (jumping, short distance running) while
"slow" muscles are for prolonged activity (body posture, marathon).

	RED SKELETAL MUSCLE	WHITE SKELETAL MUSCLE
myosin isoenzyme	slow	fast
glycolytic capacity	low	high
oxidative capacity	high	low

oxidative capacity
 related to:
• number of capillaries
• myoglobin content
• number of mitochondria

---

isotonic: force remains constant
muscle shortens during contraction

isometric: force increases during contraction
length of muscle remains constant

6.17.) ELECTROMECHANICAL COUPLING

Electromechanical coupling describes the relationship between membrane potential, intracellular Ca^{2+} and muscle contraction. There are important differences between the 3 muscle tissues:

SKELETAL MUSCLE	HEART MUSCLE	SMOOTH MUSCLE
motor units [1]	syncytium	syncytium
action potential: 2-4 ms	action potential: 200-400 ms	tonic • vascular smooth muscle phasic • visceral smooth muscle • slow waves, spikes
Ca^{2+} binds to troponin	Ca^{2+} binds to troponin	Ca^{2+} -calmodulin → MLC phosphorylation
Ca^{2+} release from SR	Ca^{2+} influx	Ca^{2+} influx and release
tetanus	no tetanus	myogenic tone

[1] *motor unit = all the muscle fibers that are innervated by one α-motoneuron*

REGULATION OF STRENGTH:

SKELETAL MUSCLE	HEART MUSCLE	SMOOTH MUSCLE
• recruitment of motor units • AP frequency	• AP duration	• membrane potential • biochemical modulation of Ca^{2+} sensitivity

6.18.) <u>CARDIAC CYCLE</u>

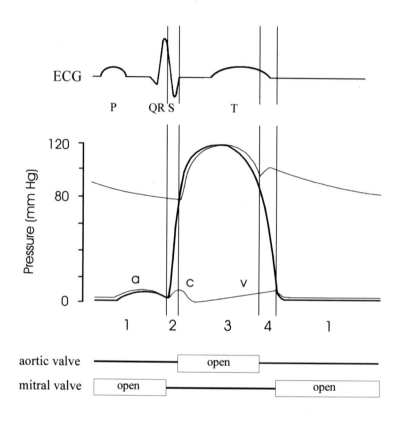

1 - filling
2 - isovolumetric contraction
3 - ejection
4 - isovolumetric relaxation

a-wave : atrial contraction
c-wave : bulging of mitral valve
v-wave : filling of atria

 All valves are closed during isovolumetric contraction or relaxation.

6.19.) LUNG VOLUMES

Lung volumes are important for diagnosis and need to be monitored in patients with restrictive or obstructive lung diseases.

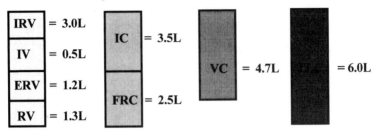

IRV	= 3.0L
IV	= 0.5L
ERV	= 1.2L
RV	= 1.3L

IC = 3.5L
FRC = 2.5L
VC = 4.7L
= 6.0L

- IRV, IV and ERV are measured by spirometer
- RV is measured by helium dilution or body plethysmography

Ventilation = dV/dt
Alveolar ventilation = ventilation - dead space ventilation

- Dead space is measured by nitrogen exhalation
  (inhale 100% oxygen, measure N_2 while exhaling)

  Dead space = anatomical dead space plus unperfused alveoli
  Ventilated alveoli that are unperfused (for example pulmonary embolism) increase dead space. This situation is called V/Q mismatch.

Ventilation / Perfusion ratio V/Q
V is higher at **base** of lung than at tip.
Q is higher at **base** of lung than at tip.
V/Q is higher at **tip** of lung than at base!

(That's why tubercle bacilli are found at tips of lung,
while pneumonia tends to develop at base of lungs.)

	OBSTRUCTIVE	RESTRICTIVE
VC	∅ or ↓	↓
FRC, RV	↑	↓
TLC	↑	↓

6.20.) <u>BREATHING PATTERNS</u>

Cheyne-Stokes		• **waxing and waning** • uremia • can be physiological at high altitude
Kussmaul		• **deep, fast inspirations** • compensation of metabolic acidosis (e.g. diabetic ketoacidosis)
Biot		• **apneic episodes** • brain tumors

Chronic lung disease (COPD):
→ central CO_2 receptors become less responsive.
→ peripheral O_2 receptors become "more important".
→ do not administer pure O_2 (patient may stop breathing!)

6.21.) <u>RESPIRATORY CENTERS</u>

EVIDENCE FROM EXPERIMENTAL TRANSSECTIONS:

IF YOU CUT:	→
above pons	normal respiration continues
above pons plus vagotomy	deeper inspirations (removal of afferent input from pulmonary sensory receptors)
mid pons	same effect as vagotomy
mid pons plus vagotomy	"apneusis" = arrested in inspiratory state [1]
below pons	irregular, fast and deep respiration (like gasping)
below medulla	all respirations seize

[1] *this finding suggests a "pneumotaxic center" located in the
rostral pons which functions to limit the extent of inspirations.*

6.22.) RESPIRATORY QUOTIENT

(CO$_2$ release / O$_2$ uptake)

RQ is a simple indicator of the metabolic status of a patient and depends on diet:

	kcal / g	RQ
carbohydrates	4	1.0
proteins	4	0.8
fat	9	0.7

RQ < 0.7	• hypoventilation • diabetes • fasting
RQ > 1.0	• hyperventilation

6.23.) ACID-BASE

How to analyze acid-base abnormalities: (1.) Check the pH to determine whether it is an acidosis or alkalosis. (2.) Check whether the main abnormality (primary disturbance) is in PCO_2 levels (respiratory) or HCO_3^- (metabolic). In clinical practice it is rare to see a "pure" abnormality, most patients have at least some degree of compensation. (3.) If you want to be more sophisticated, you can determine from published charts whether the degree of compensation matches the degree of primary disturbance. If not, you have a combined disorder.

	pH	PRIMARY DISTURBANCE	COMPENSATORY RESPONSE	CLINICAL CONDITIONS
respiratory acidosis	< 7.35	PCO_2 ↑	HCO_3^- ↑	• sedation • sleep apnea • chest wall injuries • COPD
metabolic acidosis	< 7.35	HCO_3^- ↓	PCO_2 ↓	• ketoacidosis (diabetes) • lactacidosis (shock) • chronic diarrhea
respiratory alkalosis	> 7.45	PCO_2 ↓	HCO_3^- ↓	• anxiety • thyrotoxicosis • mountain climbing
metabolic alkalosis	> 7.45	HCO_3^- ↑	PCO_2 ↑	• loop diuretics (K^+ loss) • insulin (K^+ redistribution) • vomiting (H^+ loss)

Salicylate intoxication:
Early: metabolic acidosis + respiratory alkalosis
Late: metabolic acidosis + respiratory acidosis

6.24.) HEMOGLOBINS

Hemoglobin is a protein consisting of 4 subunit chains, each containing one heme.
Heme is an iron-containing porphyrin derivative that can bind one O_2 molecule
(=oxyhemoglobin). Binding of O_2 is NOT a chemical oxidation of heme!

A) PHYSIOLOGICAL:

	HEMOGLOBIN	CHAINS
embryo	Gower 1	$\zeta_2\varepsilon_2$
fetus	HbF	$\alpha_2\gamma_2$
adult	HbA HbA$_2$ HbA$_{1C}$	$\alpha_2\beta_2$ (98%) $\alpha_2\delta_2$ (2%) glycosylated derivative

B) PATHOLOGICAL:

	HEMOGLOBIN	CHAINS
sickle cell anemia	HbS	$\alpha_2\beta^S_2$
α-thalassemia	HbH Hb Bart	β_4 γ_4
β-thalassemia	HbF HbA$_2$	$\alpha_2\delta_2$ $\alpha_2\gamma_2$

Sickle cell anemia is due to a point mutation of the β-chains. HbS
forms polymers on deoxygenation, red cells loose their deformability
and assume a sickled shape.

Hemoglobin is a major H^+ buffer of the blood. Deoxygenated hemoglobin is
less acidic than oxygenated hemoglobin and therefore ideally suited to
buffer the H^+ ions (coming from tissue CO_2) in the venous blood.

6.25.) OXYGEN BINDING CURVE

Sigmoidal relationship between PO_2 in blood and percent O_2 saturation of hemoglobin.

right shift	= **reduced binding of O_2**
	increased protons (low pH)
	increased CO_2
	increased 2,3-DPG
	increased temperature
left shift	= **tighter binding of O_2**
	fetal hemoglobin [1]
	myoglobin [1]

[1] *for a given PO_2 fetal hemoglobin and myoglobin take up more O_2. As a result, O_2 is transferred from maternal Hb to fetal Hb and from Hb to myoglobin.*

	ARTERIAL	VENOUS
PO_2	95 mmHg	40 mmHg
O_2 saturation	97 %	70 %
PCO_2	40 mmHg	45 mm Hg
pH	7.4	7.37

6.26.) BLOOD PROTEINS

serum = plasma – clotting factors

Plasma is the fluid portion of blood. If whole blood is allowed to clot and the clot is removed, the remaining fluid is called serum. Plasma proteins can be separated by size by electrophoresis:

	FUNCTIONS	DECREASED IN:
prealbumin	• thyroxine, vitamin A	
albumin	• oncotic pressure • binds hormones, drugs	• malnutrition • liver failure • pregnancy
α1 globulin	• lipoproteins • α1 antitrypsin	• α1 deficiency
α2 globulin	• haptoglobin (carries hemoglobin dimers)	• Wilson's disease
β globulin	• transferrin (carries iron)	
γ globulin	• antibodies	• agammaglobulinemia

Low levels of blood protein (liver disease, nephrotic syndrome) result in edema due to loss of oncotic pressure.

291

6.27.) CIRCULATION

Perfusion of organs is under local control. Blood flow through the brain and kidneys is autoregulated, i.e. largely independent of blood pressure. Blood flow through skeletal muscle depends on metabolites: pH, lactate, ADP...

A) PERFUSION:

perfusion (rest) (in % of cardiac output)	kidney > brain, muscle > heart
perfusion (exercise) (in % of cardiac output)	muscle >> heart > brain > kidney
specific perfusion (rest) (in ml min^{-1} / g tissue)	kidney >> heart > brain > muscle

B) PROPERTIES OF VESSELS:

largest pressure	arteries
largest resistance	arterioles
largest cross-sectional area	capillaries
largest blood volume	veins

Orthostasis (standing up):
- systolic blood pressure unchanged
- diastolic blood pressure increased
- peripheral resistance increased
- heart rate increased

6.28.) <u>FETAL CIRCULATION</u>

Fetal circulation is characterized by a R → L shunt. Oxygenated blood from the placenta passes through the right atrium and open foramen ovale into the left atrium. Deoxygenated blood from the upper body passes through the right atrium, right ventricle, pulmonary artery to the ductus arteriosus and into the aorta.

foramen ovale	right atrium → left atrium
ductus arteriosus	pulmonary artery → aorta
ductus venosus	umbilical vein → vena cava inf.

- Ductus arteriosus is kept open by prostaglandins.
- Lung maturation is accelerated by glucocorticoids.

Placenta receives 30-40% of fetal blood circulation.

Head and upper extremities (<u>preductal</u>) receive O$_2$ rich blood. Lower extremities (<u>postductal</u>) receive mixed blood.

AT BIRTH:
- Foramen ovale closes
  (left atrial pressure higher than right atrial pressure)
- Shunt reversal through ductus arteriosus L → R
  (aortic pressure higher than pulmonary artery pressure)
- Ductus arteriosus closes within a few months.

6.29.) RENAL TRANSPORT

The renal tubuli recover most of the filtered ions and small molecules and concentrate the urine to preserve water (anti-diuresis).

proximal tubule	• active resorption (glucose, amino acids etc.) • active secretion (organic acids, protons etc.) ➤ *carbonic anhydrase inhibitors act here*
Henle loop	• NaCl resorption • thick ascending portion is water impermeable! (generates osmotic gradient) ➤ *loop diuretics act here*
distal tubule	• K^+ secretion, H^+ secretion (in exchange for Na^+) ➤ *thiazide diuretics act here*
collecting duct	• water permeability under hormonal control • ADH increases permeability → water reabsorption ↑ → urine concentrated

EXCRETION OF H^+ (proximal and distal tubule):
- **Titratable acids:** H^+ (<1%), uric acid (10%), phosphate (40%)
- **Non-titratable acids:** NH_4^+ (50%)

RECOVERY OF BICARBONATE (proximal tubule):
- 99.9% of filtered HCO_3^- is recovered.
- H^+ is secreted (in exchange for Na^+) and combines with tubular HCO_3^- forming H_2CO_3 which dissociates into H_2O and CO_2. CO_2 diffuses into the cell and is split back into H^+ for secretion and HCO_3^- which then is transported through the basolateral membrane (carrier mediated) into the peritubular space.

6.30.) CLEARANCE

Clearance is the amount of plasma (per minute) that gets <u>completely</u> "cleared". If a substance is completely removed from the plasma while passing through the kidneys, then its clearance equals renal plasma flow.

	NORMAL VALUE	CALCULATED FROM MEASUREMENT OF:
RBF (renal blood flow)	1,200 mL / min	PAH clearance and hematocrit
RPF (renal plasma flow)	600 mL / min	PAH clearance
GFR (glomerular filtration rate)	125 mL / min	inulin clearance or creatinine clearance
FF (filtration fraction)	20 %	GFR / RPF

	INTERPRETATION:
clearance > GFR	filtration + net secretion
clearance = GFR	filtration only (or secretion = resorption)
clearance < GFR	filtration + net resorption

- Contraction of afferent arteriole decreases GFR.
- Contraction of efferent arteriole increases GFR.

6.31.) VOLUME REGULATION

Plasma volume and osmolarity are closely linked: The most common cause of hyperosmolarity is dehydration (loss of water)!

	RECEPTORS	MECHANISM
osmoregulation	• hypothalamus	hyperosmolarity results in: • thirst • ADH release
volume regulation	• baroreceptors • macula densa	blood volume loss results in: • sympathetic activation • renin release from JGA

6.32.) FLUID SHIFTS

	ICV	ECV	CLINICAL EXAMPLES
hypotone dehydration	↑	↓	• diarrhea, vomiting[1]
isotone dehydration	∅	↓	• blood loss
hypertone dehydration	↓	↓	• excessive sweating[2] • diabetes insipidus
hypotone hydration	↑	↑	• SIADH
isotone hydration	∅	↑	• cardiac failure • nephrotic syndrome
hypertone hydration	↓	↑	• hyperaldosteronism

[1] *loss of NaCl large compared to loss of water*
[2] *loss of water large compared to electrolytes*

6.33.) RENIN / ANGIOTENSIN

The renin-angiotensin system is the most important regulator of blood volume. It is activated when renal blood flow decreases. In cardiac failure, it results in edema and congestion.

	PRODUCED BY:	FEATURES:
angiotensinogen	liver	$\alpha 2$ globulin
((renin))	kidney (JGA)	protease
angiotensin I		
((converting enzyme))	lung	protease
angiotensin II		vasoconstriction aldosterone release
aldosterone	zona glomerulosa	Na^+ reabsorption K^+ secretion
atrial natriuretic peptide (ANP)	heart: (high ECV → stretch of atria)	natriuresis
natriuretic factor (ouabain-like inhibitor of Na^+/K^+ pump)		unknown significance

Macula densa is a modified epithelium of distal tubule, juxtaglomerular.

Renin is released when: • blood pressure at JG cells is low.
• NaCl delivery to macula densa is low.

Patients with Bartter's syndrome:
• high renin, angiotensin and aldosterone, but normotensive!
(down regulation of vascular angiotensin receptors???)

Patients with hypertension • respond to ACE inhibitors even when their renin levels are normal or low!

6.34.) INTESTINAL ABSORPTION

The digestive and absorptive functions of the GI tract are essential for life. Resection of more than 50% of the small intestine leads to malabsorption and wasting. Reduced fat absorption results in vitamin deficiencies (A,D,E and K) and bulky, greasy, foul smelling stools.

carbohydrates	duodenum	jejunum	
amino acids	duodenum	jejunum	
iron	duodenum		
vit. B12			terminal ileum
bile salts			terminal ileum

IRON:
- absorbed as Fe^{2+} (combine with anti-oxidants like vit. C)
- transported as transferrin
- stored as ferritin and hemosiderin

Defects of amino acid transporters:
- **Hartnup disease:** defect in neutral amino acid transporter
- **Cystinuria:**　　　defect in basic amino acid transporter

6.35.) GI HORMONES

The gastrointestinal tract has its own nervous system and produces hormones which regulate its digestive functions:

	RELEASED BY:	RESULTS IN:
gastrin	• vagus nerve (ACh) • peptides, alcohol and alkaline pH in stomach	• HCl secretion • increased stomach motility • delayed stomach emptying
secretin	• acidic pH in duodenum	• HCO_3^- rich pancreatic secretion
CCK	• fat and peptides in duodenum	• enzyme rich pancreatic secretion • gallbladder contractions
GIP	• glucose, fat in duodenum	• stimulates insulin secretion
somatostatin	• acidic pH in stomach	• inhibits HCl secretion (stomach) • inhibits enzyme secretion (pancreas)

6.36.) STOMACH

	MAINLY SECRETES:
chief cells [1]	• pepsinogen
parietal cells [1]	• HCl • intrinsic factor
mucus cells [1,2]	• mucus
G cells [2]	• gastrin

[1] *fundus and corpus*   [2] *antrum*

6.37.) ADRENAL HORMONES

The adrenal cortex produces 2 vital hormones plus a small amount of androgens. Overproduction or lack of these hormones results in important clinical syndromes:

	RELEASED BY:	SYNDROMES
aldosterone	• Angiotensin II • high K^+ ○ (ACTH)	**CONN** (=hyperaldosteronism) • K^+ depletion • hypertension ○ but not edematous ! ○ not hypernatremic ! • weakness, tetany **ADDISON** (hypoaldosteronism) • Na^+ loss (hypotension) • K^+ retention • H^+ retention (metabolic acidosis) • pigmentation
cortisol	• stress • ACTH	**CUSHING** (cortisol excess) • skin atrophy • muscle wasting • moon face • decreased glucose tolerance • poor wound healing • osteoporosis

Most adrenalectomized patients could survive on mineralo-corticoids alone, but would face potentially fatal hypoglycemic episodes.

6.38.) INSULIN

Insulin is an anabolic hormone with a wide range of metabolic effects:

	LIVER	MUSCLE	FAT CELLS
carbohydrates	glycogen synthesis↑ gluconeogenesis↓	glucose transport↑ glycolysis↑ glycogen synthesis↑	glucose transport↑ glycerol synthesis↑
proteins		amino acid uptake↑ protein synthesis↑	
fat	lipogenesis↑		triglyceride synthesis↑ lipolysis↓

Insulin receptor: α subunit binds insulin
β subunit has tyrosine kinase activity:
• phosphorylates itself (autophosphorylation)
• phosphorylates many other proteins
• activates ras → raf → MAP kinase cascade

6.39.) GONADOTROPE HORMONES

The gonads are under control of 2 hormones from the anterior pituitary gland. Estrogens suppress FSH (negative feedback). In infertile women, ovulation can sometimes be induced by giving an anti-estrogen.

	OVARIES	TESTES
FSH	follicle maturation	spermatogenesis
LH = ICSH	triggers ovulation luteinization of follicle	testosterone secretion (Leydig cells)

SOCIAL SCIENCES

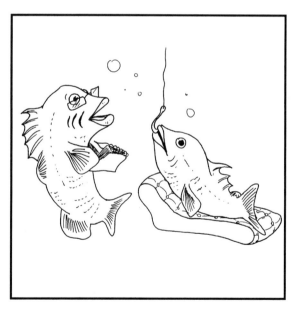

"And how long have you been feeling that
people are after you?"

Part A : Psychology

7.1.) <u>MOTOR DEVELOPMENT</u>

The nervous system continues to mature after birth. Developmental milestones are important to assess in every infant:

chin up	1 month
chest up	2 month
knee push and "swim"	6 month
sits alone / stands with help	7 month
crawls on stomach	8 month
stands holding on furniture	10 month
walks when led	11 month
stands alone	14 month
walks alone	15 month

AT THE PLAYGROUND:
- stranger anxiety: 0~1 years
- separation anxiety: 1~3 years
- parallel play: 2~3 years
- group play: 3~4 years

7.2.) PSYCHOLOGICAL DEVELOPMENT

years	Erikson	Freud	Piaget
0 - 1.5	trust vs. mistrust	oral (trust & dependence)	sensorimotor
1.5 - 3	autonomy vs. shame	anal (holding vs. letting out)	preoperational
3 - 6	initiative vs. guilt	phallic (Oedipus complex)	"
6 - 11	industry vs. inferiority	latency	concrete operational
11 - 20	identity vs. role confusion	genital (mature sexuality)	formal operational
20 - 25	intimacy vs. isolation		
25 - 50	generativity vs. stagnation		
50 - ?	integrity vs. despair		

MAJOR IDEAS:

Freud: Unconscious mental processes are the driving force motivating our behavior. Sexuality develops in stages, each stage focusing on a different body part.

Piaget: The thinking process develops in sequential stages, each stage qualitatively different from the others.

Erikson: The ego develops in stages over the entire lifetime. Each stage is characterized by a struggle that must be resolved before progressing to the next one.

7.3.) IQ TESTS

It is controversial whether intelligence is a single factor or composed of several independent factors and to what extend it is determined genetically. There is a high concordance in monozygotic twins.

Deviation Tests	Tests of Mental Age
mean: 100 standard deviation: 15 normed for each age group	IQ = mental age / biological age
WAIS adults **WISC** children **WPPSI** preschool	**Stanford Binet** (for children and teenagers)

Degrees of Mental Retardation
In most cases the cause of mental retardation remains unknown.

IQ 55 - 70 (mild)	• mentally handicapped • educable
IQ 40 - 55 (moderate)	• trainable for personal hygiene
IQ 25 - 40 (severe)	• custodial
IQ < 25 (profound)	• custodial

7.4.) CONDITIONING

Behavior can be modified through experience (=learning). Major models of learning are the "classical conditioning" (Pavlov) and "operant conditioning" (Skinner).

"CLASSICAL"	"OPERANT"
unconditioned stimulus: meat unconditioned response: salivation	operant: behavior to be modified
conditioned stimulus: bell conditioned response: salivation	positive reinforcer: candy negative reinforcer: shock primary reward: food, sex secondary reward: money, praise
• works on reflexive behavior (autonomic nervous system)	• works on autonomic nervous system or complex behavior
• reinforcement (unconditioned stimulus) occurs regardless of response	• reward / punishment depend on response
• partial reinforcement hastens extinction	• partial or variable reinforcement results in greater resistance to extinction (example: gambling addiction...)

 Extinction: Disappearance of learned behavior

7.5.) <u>DEFENSE MECHANISMS</u>

Defense mechanisms are "normal". Symptoms or disease occurs when defense mechanism break down or if the energy required to uphold the defenses becomes excessive.

- **Regression**
  Returning to immature ways of dealing with stress: crying, tantrums...
- **Repression**
  Blocking of unacceptable urges and feelings from awareness.
- **Denial**
  Blocking of unacceptable information or perceptions from awareness.
- **Rationalization**
  Substituting an acceptable motive for attitudes or behavior for an unacceptable motive.
- **Splitting**
  Maintaining a perception of others (or self) as all good or all bad.
- **Projection**
  "You are acting like a teenager, not I !"
- **Reaction formation**
  You want to 'kick his ass' but end up kissing it...
- **Isolation of affect**
  She talked about her baby's death calmly, without a sad expression.
- **Displacement**
  You are angry with your boss but shout at your kids instead.
- **Undoing**
  "Magic": knocking on wood etc.

> <u>Transference</u>
> Patient falls in love with therapist.
> <u>Countertransference</u>
> Therapist falls in love with patient.

 Always watch your countertransference !

7.6.) SLEEP STAGES

Sleep is important. Rats who are chronically deprived of sleep will die after few weeks. The role of REM sleep remains unclear. Suppression of REM sleep in volunteers appears to have no obvious ill effects.

	KEY FEATURES	EEG
awake		**beta:** > 12 / sec **alpha:** 8-12 / sec
stage 1		**theta:** 4-8 / sec
stage 2		low voltage sleep spindles
stages 3, 4	• night terrors • sleep walking • sleep talking o enuresis	**delta:** 1-4 / sec
REM	• rapid eye movements • paralysis of skeletal muscles (except eyes, finger, toes) • increased blood pressure and respiration • penis erection • dreams, nightmares	like awake state

---

Night terrors: extreme fright, no memory or dream

Narcolepsy: - patient suddenly falls asleep (REM at onset!)
- cataplexy (sudden collapse because of loss of muscle tone)
- hypnagogic hallucinations (just before falling asleep)
- sleep paralysis (awake but unable to move or speak)

Sleep apnea: central: no respiratory effort
obstructive: increased respiratory effort against
airway obstruction

7.7.) <u>SUICIDE</u>

> **<u>Risk factors:</u>** - has specific plan (always ask!)
> - lack of social support
> - recovery phase of depression
> - physicians, dentists

- success-rate: 10%
- after failed attempts: 30% will try again
- 80% have given warning

- o **women:** more overall attempts than men
- o **men:** more "successful" suicides than women
- o more common in **elderly**
- o more common in **single** than in married people
- o more common in **divorced** than in single people

LEADING CAUSES OF DEATH:

White teenagers: motor vehicle accidents > suicides > homicides
Black teenagers: homicides > motor vehicle accidents > suicides

7.8.) <u>STAGES OF DYING</u>
Elisabeth Kübler-Ross

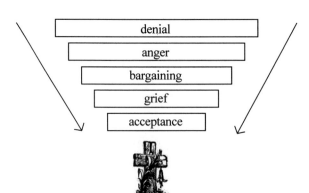

denial

anger

bargaining

grief

acceptance

Part B : Psychopathology

7.9.) NEUROTRANSMITTERS

Most major psychiatric diseases are associated with abnormal levels of neuro-transmitters. Whether these changes are the actual cause of psychiatric disease remains controversial.

	NEUROTRANSMITTER LEVELS:
schizophrenia	• dopamine ↑
depression	• norepinephrine ↓ • serotonin ↓ • dopamine ↓
Alzheimer's disease	• acetylcholine ↓ (nucleus of Meynert)
anxiety	• GABA ↓

> **Benzodiazepines and barbiturates act on GABA receptors:**
> → open Cl⁻ channels
> → hyperpolarization of nerve cell
> → decreased neuronal firing

7.10.) <u>GRIEF & DEPRESSION</u>

Grief is a normal reaction caused by loss and not reach the level of clinical depression.

GRIEF	MAJOR DEPRESSION
• initial: shock/denial • illusions / hallucinations may occur • low risk of suicide	• feeling of hopelessness • feeling of worthlessness • high risk of suicide

Abnormal grief reaction:
- *continued thoughts about guilt and death*
- *marked psychomotor retardation*
- *marked functional impairment*
- *lasts < 2 months (if longer, a diagnosis of major depression is likely)*

7.11.) <u>DELIRIUM & DEMENTIA</u>

Delirium is often caused by toxins, metabolites or infections.
Dementia most commonly is due to Alzheimer's or cerebrovascular disease.

DELIRIUM	DEMENTIA
• impaired consciousness (agitation or stupor)	• unimpaired consciousness
• develops quickly, fluctuating	• slow, progressive
• usually reversible	• irreversible

7.12.) PERSONALITY DISORDERS

Inflexible, rigid behavioral pattern that causes social impairment. Begins during adolescence and patients are usually NOT distressed and do NOT seek help.

A) ECCENTRIC:

paranoid	• patient projects his fears onto others • may blame physician or others for disease
schizoid	• anxious, withdrawn • doesn't want close relationships
schizotypal	• like schizoid PLUS odd ideas, paranoia, magical thinking • premorbid personality type of many schizophrenics

B) EMOTIONAL, DRAMATIC:

histrionic	• dramatic, emotional • may display inappropriate sexual behavior
narcissistic	• feels better than others • perfect self-image is threatened by disease
borderline	• severe disorder with features of psychoses • intense, unstable relationships • self-damaging, suicidal

C) FEARFUL, ANXIOUS:

dependent	• afraid of being helpless • need to be cared for
compulsive	• fear of loss of control • tries to control physician
avoidant	• hypersensitive to rejection or failure • fear starting relationships • strong desire for affection

7.13.) ANXIETY DISORDERS

Fear is an emotional and physiological response to a real threat, anxiety is a similar response without a clear external threat. Patients with anxiety disorders are distressed and know that their symptoms are irrational.

phobia	<ul><li>persistent excessive fear of specific objects or situations</li><li>patient knows that his fear his unrealistic</li></ul>
agoraphobia	<ul><li>history of panic attacks</li><li>patient avoids places were panic attacks might occur (especially public places)</li></ul>
obsessive-compulsive	<ul><li>**obsessions:** recurrent thoughts</li><li>**compulsions:** repetitive behavior</li></ul>
posttraumatic stress disorder	<ul><li>traumatic event in history</li><li>may occur ANY time after event</li><li>persists for > 1 month</li></ul>
generalized anxiety disorder	<ul><li>excessive anxiety and worries</li><li>restlessness, muscle tension, irritability</li></ul>

7.14.) SOMATOFORM DISORDERS

Physical symptoms without organic pathology, causing significant distress or functional impairment.

somatization
(Briquet's syndrome)
	• sickly for most of life
	• involves <u>many organ systems</u>:
	  - gastrointestinal
	  - cardiopulmonary
	  - reproductive
	  - pain
	
	• diagnosed, when at least 12 symptoms are present plus history of several years.

conversion disorder (hysterical neurosis)	• "<u>pseudo-neurological</u>" (blindness, paresthesia, paralysis) • symptoms begin and end suddenly • often misdiagnosed as "malingering"
hypochondriasis	• <u>unrealistic interpretation</u> of body signs • belief to have serious disease that goes unrecognized by family and physicians

7.15.) SCHIZOPHRENIA

Psychotic illness with disorganized thinking, speech and behavior. 1% risk among general population, 15% for persons who have a 1st degree relative with schizophrenia. Often leads to progressive mental deterioration ("dementia praecox")

positive symptoms:	• delusions • hallucinations (often auditory)
negative symptoms:	• flat affect • avolition
"four A's":	• affect inappropriate • ambivalence • associative thinking (alogical) • autism

7.16.) MAJOR DEPRESSION

Severe mood disorder that is qualitatively different from normal grief or sadness. Abnormalities in biorhythms and sleep pattern are very common in these patients.

major depression	• depressed mood • feeling of worthlessness • weight loss ! • early morning insomnia !
bipolar type 1	• at least one manic episode in patient's history
bipolar type 2	• at least one major depressive episode PLUS at least one hypomanic or manic episode

You should NOT make diagnosis of major depression within two months after bereavement (loss of a loved-one), even if the "classical" symptoms are present!

7.17.) EPILEPSY

Brief attacks of altered consciousness, motor activity and sensation caused by excessive discharge of cerebral neurons. Tonic-clonic seizures are the most common (90%).

grand mal	• tonic, then clonic • loss of consciousness • incontinence EEG : high voltage spikes
petit mal	• absence seizure ("blank spell") • no loss of muscle tone EEG : 3/sec spikes and domes
narcolepsy	• loss of muscle tone • REM onset sleep
psychomotor	• non-goal directed activity (lip smacking, walking...) EEG : spikes in temporal lobes
Jacksonian	• spreading muscle group activity (e.g. fingers → forearm → shoulder) EEG : focus around antral sulcus

7.18.) DRUG ABUSE

Abuse: Recurrent use of drugs resulting in (1.) social failures at home, school or work, (2.) legal problems (3.) hazardous situations.
Dependence: Tolerance - needs larger doses to achieve effect
- withdrawal symptoms.

	INTOXICATION	WITHDRAWAL
alcohol	• euphoria • disorientation • unsteady gait	• nausea • tremor, seizures • delusions, hallucinations • delirium tremens
barbiturates	• sedation	• can be severe! • delirium • epilepsy • coma, death
benzodiazepines	• antianxiety • sedation	• anxiety • irritability • insomnia
amphetamines, cocaine	• arousal • euphoria	• fatigue • dysphoria
opioids	• euphoria • apathy	• nausea, vomiting • sweating, fever • muscle ache
LSD	• hallucinations • anxiety • paranoid ideas	none

Blood alcohol: > 0.1% → intoxication
> 0.2% → fall asleep, anesthesia
> 0.4% → inhibition of respiration, death

Metabolic rate is 10~20 mg/dL (0.01~0.02%) per hour.

7.19.) CHILD ABUSE

More than 1 million reported cases per year in US! Abuse can be physical, emotional or sexual. Neglect is the failure to meet the child's physical or medical needs.

PHYSICAL	SEXUAL
• infants, younger children	• preadolescent, adolescents
• abuser often female	• abuser usually male
	• abuser usually known to victim
RISK FACTORS: - prematurity, low birth weight - drug abuse - parents abused as children [1] - poverty	**RISK FACTORS:** - drug abuse - single-parent home

[1] *unable to give what they never received...*

PERHAPS ACCIDENTAL	MORE LIKELY INTENTIONAL
• splash marks • injuries to front • foot soles spared	• clearly demarcated areas, no splash • injuries to back • foot soles involved
	• history of multiple injuries • retinal hemorrhage ("shaken baby")

 Report to Social Department → do not "play detective"!

Part C : Statistics

The USMLE does not require you to do complicated statistical calculations, but you need to know the definitions and when to apply which test.

7.20.) DEFINITIONS

Standard deviation: ±1s includes 68%, ±2s includes 95%, ±3s includes 99%

Mean: average value
Median: half the values are higher, half the values are lower than this
Mode: most common value
(In a perfectly symmetrical distribution, mean, median and mode are the same!)

Relative risk: (incidence with risk factor) / (incidence without risk factor)
Attributable risk: (incidence with risk factor) - (incidence without risk factor)

Chi square test. Analysis of categorical data distribution.
- *Example: Two groups of patients with chronic arthritis are given either drug or placebo. Condition after treatment will be rated "improved", "same", or "worsened".*

Paired Student's t-test. Each patient serves as its own control.
- *Example: A group of patients with hypertension is treated first with placebo then with drug (or vice versa) in a "cross-over" design.*

Correlation coefficient. Test of degree of association between two variables.
- *Example: BP and triglyceride levels are measured in a cross-sectional study of patients.*

Analysis of variance. Determine how several independent variables affect one dependent variable (similar to t-test, but more variables).
- *Example: Effect of blood pressure, cholesterol, triglycerides and patient's income on incidence of myocardial infarction.*

Analysis of covariance. Determine how several independent variables affect one dependent variable and controlling for other variables.
- *Example: Assessment of effect of drug versus placebo in two groups of patients taking pretreatment blood pressure into account.*

7.21.) <u>SENSITIVITY</u>

Sensitivity is the probability that a sick patient (A+C) will have a positive test result (A).

	patient is sick	patient is healthy
test result is positive	A	B
test result is negative	C	D

Sensitivity: divide A by (A+C)

C = "False negative"

> Tests with high sensitivity are used for screening.
> Tests with high sensitivity are used to "rule out" diagnosis.

"A test has a sensitivity of 90%" means that 10% of patients with the disease go undetected (false negative).

7.22.) <u>SPECIFICITY</u>

Specificity is the probability that a healthy patient (B+D) will have a negative test result (D).

	patient is sick	patient is healthy
test result is positive	A	B
test result is negative	C	D

Specificity: divide D by (B+D)

B = "False positive"

> ➤ Tests with high specificity are used to confirm diagnosis.

"A test has a specificity of 80%" means that 20% of people without disease get a false positive test result.

Sensitivity and specificity are <u>independent</u> of disease prevalence!

7.23.) <u>POSITIVE PREDICTIVE VALUE</u>

PPV is the probability that a patient with a positive test result (A+B) is indeed sick (A).

	patient is sick	patient is healthy
test result is positive	A	B
test result is negative	C	D

Positive predictive value: divide A by (A+B)

> ➤ The predictive value depends not only on the test's properties but also on disease prevalence.
> ➤ PPV is higher in populations with high prevalence!

If you had screened inhabitants of Siberia in 1985 for HIV antibodies, all positive results would have been false positive and the PPV would have been 0.

Screening an asymptomatic, low-risk population will result in many false positives. The expense for follow-up of false positive results (plus the alarm you cause the patient) needs to be weighed against the benefits of early disease detection.

7.24.) <u>NEGATIVE PREDICTIVE VALUE</u>

NPV is the probability that a patient with a negative test result (C+D) is indeed healthy (D).

	patient is sick	patient is healthy
test result is positive	A	B
test result is negative	C	D

Negative predictive value: divide D by (C+D)

> ➤ The predictive value depends not only on the test's properties but also on disease prevalence.
> ➤ NPV is higher in populations with low prevalence!

7.25.) CANCER STATISTICS (USA)

The most common cancer is basal cell carcinoma of the skin. Because of its low metastatic potential (<0.01%) it is not considered on "cancer statistics".

A.) Incidence

- *number of new people that develop disease in one year per 100,000 population*

MALE	FEMALE
1. prostate (41%)	1. breast (31%)
2. lung (13%)	2. lung (13%)
3. colorectal (9%)	3. colorectal (11%)

B.) Mortality

- *number of people who die of disease in one year per 100,000 population*

MALE	FEMALE
1. lung (32%)	1. lung (25%)
2. prostate (14%)	2. breast (17%)
3. colorectal (9%)	3. colon (10%)

C.) Prevalence

- *number of people who have disease at a given date (or time interval) per 100,000 population*
- *depends on both incidence and duration of disease*

7.26.) <u>RANDOMIZED CLINICAL TRIAL</u>

This is the "State of the Art" test to evaluate new drugs.

design	• researcher conducts interventions
study group	• patients are selected and assigned randomly to intervention or control groups
observation	• patients are assessed before and after intervention or control procedure

Null hypothesis:	assumes that there is no significant difference between new drug and control treatment
Type I error:	null hypothesis is rejected although it is true *(i.e. to claim that drug is effective when it is not)*
Type II error:	null hypothesis is not rejected even though it is false *(i.e. to claim that drug is not effective when it really is)*
P value:	probability of a type I error

P=0.05 means that there is a 5% probability that the observed difference between new drug and control treatment was due to chance. The lower the P value the better.

The larger the number of patients in the study, the lower P tends to be...

7.27.) OBSERVATIONAL COHORT

(prospective)

Mainly used to estimate incidence of disease in groups with different risk factors.

design	• researcher observes natural events over time • no intervention, but requires lots of time and effort
study group	• two patient groups defined by presence/absence of risk factors are compared
observation	• patients are assessed repeatedly during course of study for incidence of disease

Validity: does the test measure what it is supposed to measure?
Reliability: how well can the test results be reproduced?

Framingham Heart Study:
o sample population of Framingham, Massachusetts
o assesses risk factors for cardiovascular disease
o began in 1950, still ongoing today

7.28.) CASE CONTROL STUDY
(retrospective)

Used to identify risk factors.

design	• researcher determines presence of risk factors retrospectively
study group	• two patient groups defined by presence/absence of disease are compared
observation	• patients are assessed for presence of disease at begin of study, then questioned for risk factors

7.29.) CROSS SECTIONAL SURVEY
(convenient, common study)

Used to determine correlations between two or more variables.

design	• researcher records presence of variables • can be done on existing data base
study group	• single patient group for which association between variables is sought
observation	• data are obtained on all variables of interest at the same point of time

Correlation coefficient:	+1	perfect correlation
	0	no correlation between variables
	-1	perfect negative correlation

7.30.) LEGAL ISSUES

- **Competent patients** may refuse medical treatment, even if death will result.

- **Involuntary treatment** requires   a) patient is mentally ill
                                                        PLUS
                                                b) danger to self or others

- **Confidentiality:** May be breached if significant risk to others exists:
                                (HIV positive prostitute, patient threatens to kill, child abuse)

- **Living will:** Directions for future care (when unable to make decisions)
- **Durable power of attorney:** designate a legal representative to make decisions

---

- **Minors:** Parents must give consent
  No consent necessary if: - emergency
                                      - pregnancy
                                      - treatment of sexually transmitted diseases

- Some States require parental consent for abortion, others do not.

- Self-supporting minors are considered adults → parental consent is not required.

- **Medicare:** Care for the elderly (>65 years, part of "Social Security")
- **Medicaid:** Aid for the poor (on Welfare)

- **HMOs:**   - prepaid insurance plan
                 - physicians are paid fixed salary to take care of group of people

ABBREVIATIONS

a/w	associated with	MAC	minimal alveolar concentration
AA	amyloid associated protein	MAO	monoamine oxidase
Ab	antibodies	MHC	major histocompatibility complex
ACh	acetylcholine	MI	myocardial infarction
ADHD	attention deficit hyperactivity disorder	MIF	Müllerian inhibiting factor
AFP	alpha fetoprotein	MLC	myosin light chain
AL	amyloid light chains	MODY	maturity onset diabetes of the young
ALA	aminolevulinic acid	MS	multiple sclerosis
ANA	antinuclear antibodies	NGU	non-gonorrheal urethritis
AP	action potential	NIDDM	non insulin dependent diabetes mellitus
aPTT	partial thromboplastin time	NSAID	nonsteroidal antiinflammatory drug
ASD	atrial septal defect	PAH	p-aminohippurate
ARDS	acute respiratory distress syndrome	PAS	periodic acid Schiff reagent
BP	blood pressure	PCP	phencyclidine
CA	carcinoma	PDA	patent ductus arteriosus
CEA	carcinoembryonic antigen	PDE	phosphodiesterase
CoA	coenzyme A	PG	prostaglandin
COPD	chronic obstructive pulmonary disease	PMN	polymorph nuclear leukocyte
CSF	cerebrospinal fluid	PT	prothrombin time
CNS	central nervous system	RBC	red blood cells
DES	diethylstilbestrol	RSV	respiratory syncytial virus
DIC	disseminated intravascular coagulation	SLE	systemic lupus erythematosus
DOC	drug of choice	ss	single stranded
ds	double stranded	SSPE	subacute sclerosing panencephalitis
DX	differential diagnosis	TCA	tricyclic antidepressants
EBV	Epstein-Barr virus	THC	tetrahydrocannabinol
ECV	extracellular volume	TIA	transient ischemic attack
EEE	eastern equine encephalitis	TLC	total lung capacity
G6PD	glucose-6-phosphate dehydrogenase	TPA	tissue plasminogen activator
GABA	gamma-aminobutyrate	TRAP	tartrate resistant alkaline phosphatase
GBM	glomerular basement membrane	TT	thrombin time
GH	growth hormone	TX	treatment
GI	gastrointestinal	UMN	upper motor neuron
GN	glomerulonephritis	UTI	urinary tract infection
HCG	human chorionic gonadotropin	VD	venereal disease
IDDM	insulin dependent diabetes mellitus	VDRL	Venereal Disease Research Laboratory
JGA	juxtaglomerular apparatus	VSD	ventricular septal defect
LMN	lower motor neuron	VZV	varicella zoster virus
LSD	lysergic acid diethylamide	WEE	western equine encephalitis

INDEX

Benztropine, 3.50
Berger's disease, 1.47
Berry aneurysms, 1.13
Beta-agonists, 3.28, 3.35
Beta-blockers, 3.19, 3.35
Beta-lactamase, 3.7
Beta-receptors, 6.13
Bethanechol, 3.37
Bicarbonate, 6.1, 6.29
Bile acids, **4.15**
Biot respiration, 6.20
Biperiden, 3.50
Bipolar disorder, 7.16
Bismuth, 3.34
Bladder, urinary, 3.37
Blastomycosis, 2.31
Bleeding disorders, **1.22**
Bleomycin, 3.14, 3.16
Blood alcohol, 7.18
Blood pressure, 6.11
Blood proteins, **6.26**
Bone diseases, **1.72**
Bone marrow suppression, 3.3
Bone tumors, **1.74**
Borderline personality, 7.12
Bordetella, 2.16
Bornholm disease, 2.24
Borrelia burgdorferi, 2.19
Botulinum toxin, 2.4
Botulism, 2.12
Bovine spongiform encephalopathy, 2.27
Bowel infarction, 5.20
Bowen's disease, 1.87
Brachial plexus, **5.12, 5.13, 5.14**
Brain tumors, **1.76**
Brainstem syndromes, **5.33 - 5.36**
Branchial arches, **5.3**
BRCA, 1.55
Breast diseases, **1.55**
Breathing patterns, **6.20**
Bretylium, 3.27
Briquet's syndrome, 7.14
Broca, 5.24
Bromocriptine, 3.21, 3.50

Bronchiectasis, 1.43
Bronchitis, 1.43, 2.6
Bronchopneumonia, 1.45
Brucella, 2.15
Bruton's agammaglobulinemia, 1.14, 1.21
Burkitt lymphoma, 1.7, 1.29, 2.23
Buspirone, 3.46
Butyrophenone, 3.51

C
C. donovani, 1.50
Cadmium, 1.89
Caffeine, 3.45
Calcium channel blockers, 3.19
Calories, 4.24
cAMP, 6.4
Campylobacter jejuni, 2.14, 3.6
Cancer statistics, **7.25**
Candida, 1.50, 2.31, 3.6, 3.10, 3.12
Captopril, 3.20
Carbachol, 3.37
Carbamazepine, 3.52
Carbenicillin, 3.7
Carbidopa, 3.50
Carbinoxamine, 3.48
Carbon monoxide, 3.4
Carbonic anhydrase inhibitors, 3.22
Carcinoid, 1.46
Cardiac cycle, **6.18**
Cardiac index, 6.1
Cardiac output, 6.1
Cardiolipin, 4.16
Carpal tunnel syndrome, 5.14
Cartilage, **1.73**
Case control studies, **7.28**
Castor oil, 3.54
Cat bites, 2.15
Catabolic, 4.39
Catalase, 2.7
Cataplexy, 7.6
Cauda equina lesion, 5.36
CCK, 6.35
CEA, 1.9
Cefamandole, 3.8
Cefazolin, 3.8

Ethacrynic acid, 3.22
Ethosuximide, 3.52
Ethylene glycol, 3.4
Eunuchoid, 1.80
Ewing's sarcoma, 1.74
Exfoliatin, 2.7
Exonuclease, 4.45
Exotoxins, 2.4, 2.7, 2.8
Exudation, 1.1
Eye, **5.7**

F
Fabry disease, 1.14, 4.18
Facilitated transport, 6.3
Fallot's tetralogy, 1.36
Familial hypercholesterolemia, 1.13
Familial polyposis, 1.13, 1.60
Famotidine, 3.34
Fanconi anemia, 1.24
Farsightedness, 6.7
Fasting, 4.22
Fatty acids, **4.14**
Febrile seizures, 3.52
Felty's syndrome, 1.26, 1.71
Femur neck fractures, 5.16
Fentanyl, 3.42
Fetal alcohol syndrome, 1.36
Fetal circulation, **6.28**
Fetal hydantoin syndrome, 1.36
Fetal remnants, **5.2**
Fever, 1.1
Fibers, 3.54
Fibroadenoma, 1.55
Fibrocystic change, 1.55
Fibrosis of lung, 1.44
Filtration fraction, 6.30
Flecainide, 3.27
Flora, normal, **2.2**
Flukes, **2.36**
Fluorouracil, 3.14, 4.42
Fluoxetine, 3.43
Fluphenazine, 3.51
Food poisoning, 1.17
Foot drop, 5.18
Foramen magnum, 5.6

Foramen ovale, 5.6, 6.28
Foramen rotundum, 5.6
Foramen spinosum, 5.6
Fragile X, 1.14
Framingham heart study, 7.27
Francisella, 2.15
Frank Starling mechanism, 6.14
Freud, 7.2
Friedreich's ataxia, 1.77
Fructose intolerance, 4.9, 4.10
Fructosuria, 4.9
FSH, 6.39
Fungal diseases, **2.31**, 3.10
Fungi, **2.30**
Furanose, 4.6
Furosemide, 3.22

G
G proteins, **6.4**
G6PD deficiency, 1.14, 1.23, 3.3
Galactosemia, 4.9, 4.10
Gallbladder carcinoma, **1.64**
Ganciclovir, 3.9
Gardner's syndrome, 1.60
Gastric ulcer, 3.6
Gastrin, 6.35
Gastritis, **1.58**
Gastroenteritis, **1.59**
Gastrointestinal hormones, **6.35**
Gaucher's disease, 4.18
Gene expression, **4.43**
Genetics of disease, **1.11**
Genital herpes, 1.50
Germ cell tumors, 1.51
Germ layers, **5.1**
German measles, 2.24
Gestational diabetes, 1.85
Ghon complex, 2.17
Giant cell arteritis, 1.33
Giardia lamblia, 2.34
Giemsa, 2.1
Gilbert's syndrome, 1.65
GIP, 6.35
Glioblastoma, 1.76

HLA, **1.16**
HMOs, 7.30
Hodgkin's disease, 1.29, 3.16
Homocystinuria, 4.4, 4.5
Horner's syndrome, 5.7
Howell-Jolly bodies, 1.25
HPV, 1.50
HSV, 1.50, 2.23
Humerus fracture, 5.14
Hunter syndrome, 4.13
Huntington's disease, 1.13, 1.77, 5.31
Hurler syndrome, 4.13
Hutchinson's teeth, 1.36
Hydatidiform mole, 1.54
Hydrochlorothiazide, 3.22
Hydroxysteroids, 4.28
Hyperlipidemia, **3.32, 3.33**
Hypermetropia, 6.7
Hypersensitivity, **1.6**
Hypersensitivity arteritis, 1.33
Hypersensitivity pneumonitis, 1.44
Hypertension, 1.17
Hypnagogic hallucinations, 7.6
Hypnotic drugs, **3.47**
Hypochondriasis, 7.14
Hypoglossal canal, 5.6
Hypoglossal nerve, 5.8
Hypoglycemic reaction, 3.30
Hysterical neurosis, 7.14
Ibuprofen, 3.17

I
ICSH, 6.39
IDDM, 1.16, 1.85
Idoxuridine, 3.9
IgA deficiency, 1.21
Immunodeficiencies, **1.21**
Impetigo, 1.88
Incidence, 7.25
India ink, 2.1
Indomethacin, 3.17
Inducers, 4.43
Infectious mononucleosis, 2.23
Inflammation, **1.1**

Inflammatory bowel disease, **1.61**
Influenza, 2.24
Inotropic drugs, **3.28**
Insulin, **3.30**, 4.39, **6.38**
Insulin receptor, 6.38
Interferon, 3.9
Internal carotid artery, 5.27
Intestinal absorption, **6.34**
Ion channels, **6.2**
IP3, 6.4
IQ tests, **7.3**
Iron, 3.4, 6.34
Iron deficiency anemia, 1.24
Ischemic heart disease, **1.37**
Isoflurane, 3.49
Isolation of affect, 7.5
Isometric contraction, 6.16
Isoniazid, 1.68
Isoproterenol, 3.35
Isosorbide dinitrate, 3.23
Isotonic contraction, 6.16
Isotretinoin, 1.36
ITP, 1.22
Itraconazole, 3.10

J
Jacksonian seizures, 7.17
Janeway lesions, 1.40
Jaundice, **1.65**
Jugular foramen, 5.6
Juvenile rheumatoid arthritis, 1.16

K
Kala-Azar, 2.33
Kaposi sarcoma, 2.23
Kartagener's, 1.43
Kawasaki, 1.33
Keratoacanthoma, 1.87
Ketamine, 3.49
Ketoconazole, 3.10
Ketogenic, 4.2
Ketosteroids, 4.28
Key enzymes, **4.25, 4.26, 4.27**
Klebsiella, 2.13

Natriuretic factor, 6.33
Nearsightedness, 6.7
Necator, 2.38
Negative predictive value, **7.24**
Neisseria, **2.9**
Nematodes, **2.38**
Neostigmine, 3.35
Nephritic syndrome, 1.17, 1.47
Nephrotic syndrome, 1.17, 1.47
Nernst equation, 6.2
Nerve fibers, **6.5**
Neural Crest, 1.76, 5.1
Neural Tube, 1.76, 5.1
Neuroblastoma, 1.81
Neurofibroma, 1.76
Neurolept anesthesia, 3.49
Neuroleptics, **3.51**
Neuromuscular block, 3.39
Neurotransmitters, **7.9**
Neutropenia, **1.26**
Neutrophilia, 1.27
Niacin, 3.33, 4.3
Nicotine, 3.45
Nicotinic antagonists, **3.39**
Nicotinic receptors, 6.12
NIDDM, 1.85
Niemann-Pick disease, 4.18
Nifedipine, 3.23
Nifurtimox, 3.11
Night terrors, 7.6
Nitroglycerin, 3.23
Nitrous oxide, 3.49
Nocardia, 2.18
Non-Hodgkin lymphoma, 1.29, 1.7
Normal flora, **2.2**
NSAIDs, **3.17**
Nucleotides, **4.40**
Null hypothesis, 7.26
Nystagmus, **6.8**
Nystatin, 3.10

O
Observational cohort, **7.27**
Obsessive compulsive, 7.13
Obstructive lung disease, **1.43**

Okazaki fragments, 4.45
Oligoclonal bands, 1.78
Oligodendroblastoma, 1.76
Omeprazole, 3.34
Onchocerca, 2.38
Oncogenes, **1.7**
Oncoviruses, 2.28
Operant conditioning, 7.4
Operator, 4.43
Operon, 4.43
Opiates, 3.4, 7.18, **3.42**
Optic canal, 5.6
Oral contraceptives, 3.40
Orbital fissure, 5.6
Organophosphates, 3.4, 3.36
Orthostasis, 6.27
Osler nodes, 1.40
Osmic acid, 2.1
Osmoregulation, **6.31**
Osmotic diuretics, 3.22
Osteoarthritis, 1.71
Osteoblastoma, 1.74
Osteochondroma, 1.73
Osteogenesis imperfecta, 1.72
Osteoid osteoma, 1.74
Osteoma, 1.74
Osteomalacia, 1.72
Osteomyelitis, 3.6
Osteopetrosis, 1.72
Osteoporosis, 1.72
Osteosarcoma, 1.74
Otitis media, 2.6
Ototoxicity, 3.3
Ovarian tumors, **1.52**
Ovaries, 5.24, **4.32, 4.33**
Ovulation, 6.39
Oxygen binding curve, **6.25**

P
p value, 7.26
p24, 2.29
p53, 1.8
Pacinian corpuscle, 6.6
Paget's disease, 1.55, 1.72
Pain, 1.1

Pancuronium, 3.39
Papilloma, 1.55
Papovavirus, 2.22
Paradoxical cold, 6.6
Paragonimus, 2.36
Parallel play, 7.1
Paraneoplastic syndromes, 1.46
Paranoid personality, 7.12
Parasympathetic ganglia, **5.30**
Parasympathetic nerves, 6.11
Parathyroids, **1.84**
Parietal cells, 6.36
Parkinson's disease, 1.77, **3.50**, 5.31
Parvovirus, 2.22
PAS, 2.1
Passive-aggressive personality, 7.12
Pasteurella, 2.15
Patent ductus arteriosus, 1.35, 1.36
Pedigrees, **1.11**
Pellagra, 4.4
Pelvic fractures, 5.16
Pelvic inflammatory disease, 3.6
Pemphigoid, 1.88
Pemphigus, 1.88
Penicillins, **3.7**
Pentazocine, 3.42
Pentoses, 4.6
Peptic ulcer, **3.34**
Peptide bond, 4.2
Perfusion, 6.27
Pericarditis, **1.41**
Peripheral neuropathy, 5.36
Peripheral vascular resistance, 6.1
Peritoneum, **5.22**
Peritonitis, 5.22
Peroneal nerve, 5.18
Personality disorders, **7.12**
Pertussis toxin, 2.16
Petit mal, 3.52, 7.17
Peutz-Jeghers, 1.60
Phacomatoses, 1.13
Phagocytosis, 1.1
Pharyngeal clefts, 5.3
Pharyngeal pouches, **5.4**
Pharyngitis, 2.6, 3.6

Phencyclidine, 3.41
Phenobarbital, 3.47, 3.52
Phenothiazine, 3.51
Phenoxybenzamine, 3.35
Phentolamine, 3.35
Phenylbutazone, 3.17
Phenylephrine, 3.35
Phenylketonuria, 1.12, 4.4, 4.5
Phenytoin, 3.27, 3.52
Pheochromocytoma, 1.81
Philadelphia chromosome, 1.28
Phlebothrombosis, **1.31**
Phobia, 7.13
Phosphodiesterase inhibitors, 3.28, 6.4
Phospholipids, **4.16**
Photosensitivity, 3.3, 4.20
Physical abuse, 7.19
Physostigmine, 3.36
Piaget, 7.2
Pick's disease, 1.77
Picorna virus, 2.24
Pilocarpine, 3.37
Pindolol, 3.35
Pirenzepine, 3.34
Pituitary, **1.79**, **1.80**
Pityriasis, 1.88
Placenta, **1.54**
Plague, 2.15, 3.6
Plasma cell neoplasia, **1.30**
Platelet aggregation inhibitors, **3.24**
Play, 7.1
Plummer's disease, 1.82
Plummer-Vinson syndrome, 1.24
Pneumoconiosis, 1.44
Pneumocystis carinii, 2.33, 3.12
Pneumonia, **1.45**, 2.6, 3.6
Pneumotaxic center, 6.21
Poliomyelitis, 2.24
Polyarteritis nodosa, 1.33
Polycystic renal disease, 1.12, 1.13
Polymerase, 4.44
Polyposis, 1.13, **1.60**
Polysaccharides, **4.8**
Pompe's disease, 4.11

Replication, inhibitors of, **3.14**
Repression, 7.5
Repressor, 4.43
Reserpine, 3.35
Respiratory centers, **6.21**
Respiratory quotient, **6.22**
Restrictive lung diseases, **1.44**
Reticulocytes, 1.25
Retinoblastoma, 1.8, 1.15
Retroperitoneum, 5.22
Retroviruses, **2.28**
Reverse transcriptase, 2.29
Reye's syndrome, 3.17
Rheumatic fever, **1.42**
Rheumatic heart disease, **1.42**
Rheumatoid arthritis, 1.4, 1.16, 1.71
Ribavirin, 3.9
Rickettsia, **2.21**
Riedel's struma, 1.82
Rifampin, 3.15
Rinne test, 6.10
River blindness, 2.38
RNA viruses, **2.24**
Rocky Mountain spotted fever, 2.21
Rofecoxib, 3.17
Rosacea, 1.88
Roseola, 2.23
Rotator cuff, 5.11
Rotavirus, 2.24
Roth spots, 1.40
Rotor syndrome, 1.65
Roundworms, 2.38
Rubella, 2.24
Rubeola, 2.24

S
Saccharide, **4.8**
Saccharide disorders, **4.9**
Salicylate intoxication, 3.17, 6.23
Salmon patches, 1.88
Salmonella, 2.13
Salt retention, 4.38
Salt wasting, 4.37

Saralasin, 3.20
Scapular winging, 5.11
Scheie syndrome, 4.13
Schilder's disease, 1.78
Schistosoma, 2.36
Schizoid personality, 7.12
Schizophrenia, **7.15**
Schwannoma, 1.76
Scopolamine, 3.38
Scrapie, 2.27
Seborrheic keratosis, 1.87
Secretin, 6.35
Seminoma, 1.51
Senna, 3.54
Sensitivity, **7.21**
Separation anxiety, 7.1
Sepsis, 2.6, 3.6
Sertoli cells, 1.51
Serum sickness, 1.6
Sex hormones, **3.40**
Sexual abuse, 7.19
Sheehan's syndrome, 1.80
Shigella, 2.13
Shingles, 2.23
Shoulder, **5.11**
Sick euthyroid, 1.82
Sickle cell anemia, 1.12, 1.23, 6.24
Side effects, **3.3**
Siderocytes, 1.25
Sigma factor, 4.44
Signal transduction, **6.4**
Sinusitis, 2.6
Sjögren's syndrome, **1.20**
Skeletal muscle, **6.17**
Skin cancer, **1.87**
Skin diseases, **1.88**
Skin infections, 3.10
Skull, **5.6**
SLE, 1.4, 1.16, **1.18**
Sleep apnea, 7.6
Sleep stages, **7.6**
Sleep walking, 7.6
Sleeping sickness, 2.33, 3.11
Slow viral diseases, **2.26**

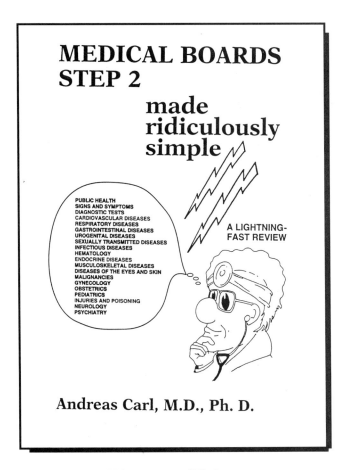

MEDICAL BOARDS STEP 2

made ridiculously simple

PUBLIC HEALTH
SIGNS AND SYMPTOMS
DIAGNOSTIC TESTS
CARDIOVASCULAR DISEASES
RESPIRATORY DISEASES
GASTROINTESTINAL DISEASES
UROGENITAL DISEASES
SEXUALLY TRANSMITTED DISEASES
INFECTIOUS DISEASES
HEMATOLOGY
ENDOCRINE DISEASES
MUSCULOSKELETAL DISEASES
DISEASES OF THE EYES AND SKIN
MALIGNANCIES
GYNECOLOGY
OBSTETRICS
PEDIATRICS
INJURIES AND POISONING
NEUROLOGY
PSYCHIATRY

A LIGHTNING-
FAST REVIEW

Andreas Carl, M.D., Ph. D.

356 pages - 273 charts

♦ All the Facts about Diseases and Organ Systems in Chart Format
♦ "Hot-Lists" cover Patient Management and Therapy

MEDICAL BOARDS STEP 3

made ridiculously simple

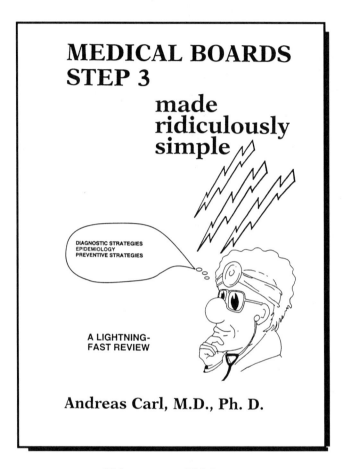

DIAGNOSTIC STRATEGIES
EPIDEMIOLOGY
PREVENTIVE STRATEGIES

A LIGHTNING-
FAST REVIEW

Andreas Carl, M.D., Ph. D.

286 pages - 394 charts

- A Step-by-Step Approach (*"what to do next ?"*)
- Diagnosis and Management of Diseases